Quality of Care and Information Technology

Editor

SRINIVASAN SURESH

PEDIATRIC CLINICS OF NORTH AMERICA

www.pediatric.theclinics.com

Consulting Editor
BONITA F. STANTON

April 2016 • Volume 63 • Number 2

ELSEVIER

1600 John F. Kennedy Boulevard • Suite 1800 • Philadelphia, Pennsylvania, 19103-2899

http://www.theclinics.com

THE PEDIATRIC CLINICS OF NORTH AMERICA Volume 63, Number 2
April 2016 ISSN 0031-3955, ISBN-13: 978-0-323-41765-5

Editor: Kerry Holland
Developmental Editor: Casey Jackson

The Pediatric Clinics of North America (ISSN 0031-3955) is published bimonthly by Elsevier Inc., 360 Park Avenue South, New York, NY 10010-1710. Months of issue are February, April, June, August, October, and December. Periodicals postage paid at New York, NY and additional mailing offices. Subscription prices are $200.00 per year (US individuals), $556.00 per year (US institutions), $270.00 per year (Canadian individuals), $740.00 per year (Canadian institutions), $325.00 per year (international individuals), $740.00 per year (international institutions), $100.00 per year (US students and residents), and $165.00 per year (international and Canadian residents and students). To receive students/resident rare, orders must be accompanied by name of affiliated institution, date of term, and the signature of program/residency coordinator on institution letterhead. Orders will be billed at individual rate until proof of status is received. Foreign air speed delivery is included in all *Clinics* subscription prices. All prices are subject to change without notice. **POSTMASTER:** Send address changes to *The Pediatric Clinics of North America*, Elsevier Health Sciences Division, Subscription Customer Service, 3251 Riverport Lane, Maryland Heights, MO 63043. **Customer Service: 1-800-654-2452 (US and Canada). From outside of the US and Canada: 1-314-447-8871. Fax: 1-314-447-8029. For print support, E-mail: JournalsCustomerService-usa@elsevier.com. For online support, E-mail: JournalsOnlineSupport-usa@elsevier.com.**

Reprints. For copies of 100 or more, of articles in this publication, please contact the Commercial Reprints Department, Elsevier Inc., 360 Park Avenue South, New York, NY 10010-1710. Tel.: 212-633-3874; Fax: 212-633-3820; E-mail: reprints@elsevier.com.

The Pediatric Clinics of North America is also published in Spanish by McGraw-Hill Inter-americana Editores S.A., Mexico City, Mexico; in Portuguese by Riechmann and Affonso Editores, Rua Comandante Coelho 1085, CEP 21250, Rio de Janeiro, Brazil; and in Greek by Althayia SA, Athens, Greece.

The Pediatric Clinics of North America is covered in *MEDLINE/PubMed (Index Medicus), Excerpta Medica, Current Contents, Current Contents/Clinical Medicine, Science Citation Index, ASCA, ISI/BIOMED,* and *BIOSIS.*

PROGRAM OBJECTIVE

The goal of the *Pediatric Clinics of North America* is to keep practicing physicians and residents up to date with current clinical practice in pediatrics by providing timely articles reviewing the state-of-the-art in patient care.

TARGET AUDIENCE

All practicing pediatricians, physicians and healthcare professionals who provide patient care to pediatric patients.

LEARNING OBJECTIVES

Upon completion of this activity, participants will be able to:
1. Review patient safety measures in pediatric medicine.
2. Discuss considerations in the improvement of clinical effectiveness and quality improvement in pediatric medicine.
3. Recognize the opportunities and challenges of using telehealth and advanced technology in pediatric settings.

ACCREDITATION

The Elsevier Office of Continuing Medical Education (EOCME) is accredited by the Accreditation Council for Continuing Medical Education (ACCME) to provide continuing medical education for physicians.

The EOCME designates this enduring material for a maximum of 15 *AMA PRA Category 1 Credit*(s)™. Physicians should claim only the credit commensurate with the extent of their participation in the activity.

All other health care professionals requesting continuing education credit for this enduring material will be issued a certificate of participation.

DISCLOSURE OF CONFLICTS OF INTEREST

The EOCME assesses conflict of interest with its instructors, faculty, planners, and other individuals who are in a position to control the content of CME activities. All relevant conflicts of interest that are identified are thoroughly vetted by EOCME for fair balance, scientific objectivity, and patient care recommendations. EOCME is committed to providing its learners with CME activities that promote improvements or quality in healthcare and not a specific proprietary business or a commercial interest.

The planning committee, staff, authors and editors listed below have identified no financial relationships or relationships to products or devices they or their spouse/life partner have with commercial interest related to the content of this CME activity:

Erika Abramson, MD, MS, FAAP; Andrew R. Buchert, MD; Gabriella A. Butler, MSN, RN; N. Lance Downing, MD; Anjali Fortna; Sean A. Frederick, MD; Veena V. Goel, MD; Kerry Holland; Diane S. Hupp, DNP, RN, NEA-BC; David C. Kaelber, MD, PhD, MPH; Bhanumathy Kumar, MD, FAAP; Indu Kumari; Christopher A. Longhurst, MD, MS; Brian S. Martin, DMD, MHCDS; Emily Mathias, MD; Matthew F. Niedner, MD; Johanna R. Rosen, MD; Richard A. Saladino, MD; Usha Sethuraman, MD; Bonita F. Stanton, MD; Megan Suermann; Srinivasan Suresh, MD, MBA, FAAP; Scott M. Sutherland, MD; Levon Utidjian, MD, FAAP; Emily C. Webber, MD.

UNAPPROVED/OFF-LABEL USE DISCLOSURE

The EOCME requires CME faculty to disclose to the participants:
1. When products or procedures being discussed are off-label, unlabelled, experimental, and/or investigational (not US Food and Drug Administration [FDA] approved); and
2. Any limitations on the information presented, such as data that are preliminary or that represent ongoing research, interim analyses, and/or unsupported opinions. Faculty may discuss information about pharmaceutical agents that is outside of FDA-approved labelling. This information is intended solely for CME and is not intended to promote off-label use of these medications. If you have any questions, contact the medical affairs department of the manufacturer for the most recent prescribing information.

TO ENROLL

To enroll in the *Pediatric Clinics of North America* Continuing Medical Education program, call customer service at 1-800-654-2452 or sign up online at http://www.theclinics.com/home/cme. The CME program is available to subscribers for an additional annual fee of USD 290.

METHOD OF PARTICIPATION

In order to claim credit, participants must complete the following:

1. Complete enrolment as indicated above.
2. Read the activity.
3. Complete the CME Test and Evaluation. Participants must achieve a score of 70% on the test. All CME Tests and Evaluations must be completed online.

CME INQUIRIES/SPECIAL NEEDS

For all CME inquiries or special needs, please contact elsevierCME@elsevier.com.

Contributors

CONSULTING EDITOR

BONITA F. STANTON, MD
Vice Dean for Research and Professor of Pediatrics, School of Medicine, Wayne State University, Detroit, Michigan

EDITOR

SRINIVASAN SURESH, MD, MBA, FAAP
Chief Medical Information Officer, Children's Hospital of Pittsburgh of UPMC, Visiting Professor of Pediatrics, University of Pittsburgh School of Medicine, Pittsburgh, Pennsylvania

AUTHORS

ERIKA ABRAMSON, MD, MS, FAAP
Assistant Professor, Department of Pediatrics; Assistant Professor, Healthcare Policy and Research, Weill Cornell Medicine, New York, New York

ANDREW R. BUCHERT, MD
Medical Director, Clinical Resource Management and Education Outreach, Children's Hospital of Pittsburgh of UPMC; Associate Medical Director for GME Quality and Safety, Donald D Wolff Center for Quality, Safety, and Innovation; Assistant Professor of Pediatrics, University of Pittsburgh School of Medicine, Pittsburgh, Pennsylvania

GABRIELLA A. BUTLER, MSN, RN
Manager, Clinical Resource Management, Solutions for Patient Safety, Clinical Quality Analytics, Children's Hospital of Pittsburgh of UPMC, Pittsburgh, Pennsylvania

N. LANCE DOWNING, MD
Clinical Informatics Fellow, Department of Clinical Informatics, Stanford Children's Health, Stanford, California

SEAN A. FREDERICK, MD
University of Pittsburgh Medical Center Newborn Medicine Program, Assistant Chief Medical Information Officer, Children's Hospital of Pittsburgh of UPMC, Assistant Professor of Pediatrics, University of Pittsburgh School of Medicine, Pittsburgh, Pennsylvania

VEENA V. GOEL, MD
Clinical Informatics Fellow, Department of Pediatrics, Stanford University School of Medicine; Department of Clinical Informatics, Stanford Children's Health, Stanford, California

DIANE S. HUPP, DNP, RN, NEA-BC
Vice President, Patient Care Services; Chief Nursing Officer, Children's Hospital of Pittsburgh of UPMC, Pittsburgh, Pennsylvania

DAVID C. KAELBER, MD, PhD, MPH
Professor, Departments of Information Services, Internal Medicine, Pediatrics, Epidemiology and Biostatistics, Center for Clinical Informatics Research and Education, The MetroHealth System, Case Western Reserve University, Cleveland, Ohio

BHANUMATHY KUMAR, MD, FAAP
Assistant Professor, Department of Pediatrics, Children's Hospital of Michigan, Wayne State University, Detroit, Michigan

CHRISTOPHER A. LONGHURST, MD, MS
Clinical Professor, Department of Biomedical Informatics, University of California San Diego School of Medicine, San Diego, California

BRIAN S. MARTIN, DMD, MHCDS
Medical Director-Clinical Excellence, Chief-Division of Pediatric Dentistry, Children's Hospital of Pittsburgh of UPMC, Pittsburgh, Pennsylvania

EMILY MATHIAS, MD
Fellow Physician, Pediatric Emergency Medicine, Carman and Ann Adams Department of Pediatrics, Wayne State University, Detroit, Michigan

MATTHEW F. NIEDNER, MD
Director of Quality Improvement and Patient Safety, Pediatric Intensive Care Unit, Assistant Professor, Department of Pediatrics, Division of Pediatric Critical Care Medicine, Mott Children's Hospital, University of Michigan Medical Center, Ann Arbor, Michigan

JOHANNA R. ROSEN, MD
Assistant Professor of Pediatrics, University of Pittsburgh School of Medicine, Division of Pediatric Emergency Medicine, Department of Pediatrics, Children's Hospital of Pittsburgh, UPMC, Pittsburgh, Pennsylvania

RICHARD A. SALADINO, MD
Professor of Pediatrics, University of Pittsburgh School of Medicine, Division of Pediatric Emergency Medicine, Department of Pediatrics, Children's Hospital of Pittsburgh, University of Pittsburgh Medical Center, Pittsburgh, Pennsylvania

USHA SETHURAMAN, MD
Associate Professor, Fellowship Program Director, Pediatric Emergency Medicine, Carman and Ann Adams Department of Pediatrics, Wayne State University, Detroit, Michigan

SRINIVASAN SURESH, MD, MBA, FAAP
Chief Medical Information Officer, Children's Hospital of Pittsburgh of UPMC, Visiting Professor of Pediatrics, University of Pittsburgh School of Medicine, Pittsburgh, Pennsylvania

SCOTT M. SUTHERLAND, MD
Clinical Associate Professor, Department of Pediatrics, Stanford University School of Medicine; Department of Clinical Informatics, Stanford Children's Health, Stanford, California

LEVON UTIDJIAN, MD, MBI, FAAP
Clinical Instructor, Department of Pediatrics, The Children's Hospital of Philadelphia, Perelman School of Medicine at the University of Pennsylvania; Member, Department of Biomedical and Health Informatics, The Children's Hospital of Philadelphia, Philadelphia, Pennsylvania

EMILY C. WEBBER, MD
Associate Professor of Clinical Pediatrics, Indiana University School of Medicine; Medical Director for Pediatric Informatics, IU Health; Affiliated Scientist, Regenstrief Institute, Center for Biomedical Informatics; Indianapolis, Indiana

Contents

> Applications of health information technology (health IT) are now wide-spread in the form of electronic medical records (EMRs), greatly reshaping the practice of clinical pediatrics. Population health stands to benefit greatly from the data produced by the alignment of pediatrics with other social determinants of health: medical care, genetics, individual behavior, social and physical environment. Before this potential can be realized, population health information models must be integrated into the design and evolution of EMRs and other data sources.

> Peer-to-peer benchmarking is an important component of rapid-cycle performance improvement in patient safety and quality-improvement efforts. Institutions should carefully examine critical success factors before engagement in peer-to-peer benchmarking in order to maximize growth and change opportunities. Solutions for Patient Safety has proven to be a high-yield engagement for Children's Hospital of Pittsburgh of University of Pittsburgh Medical Center, with measureable improvement in both organizational process and culture.

> Initially described more than 50 years ago, electronic health records (EHRs) are now becoming ubiquitous throughout pediatric health care settings. The confluence of increased EHR implementation and the exponential growth of digital data within them, the development of clinical informatics tools and techniques, and the growing workforce of experienced EHR users presents new opportunities to use EHRs to augment clinical discovery and improve pediatric patient care. This article reviews the basic concepts surrounding EHR-enabled research and clinical

patient safety. Best practices for incorporating quality improvement and patient safety into the curriculum of residents and fellows remains an area of interest for educators.

Health care in the United States is plagued by errors, inconsistencies, and inefficiencies. It is also extremely costly. Clinical pathways can drive high-value care and high reliability within a health care organization. Clinical pathways are much more than just guidelines or order sets as a part of a protocol of care, however; they must incorporate multiple elements that are critical to their successful implementation and sustainability. Additionally, clinical pathways can be utilized to accomplish strategic goals of the organization while fulfilling the quality, safety, and clinical aspects of the organization's mission.

Patient safety and quality are 2 of many competing priorities facing health care providers. As safety and quality rise on the agenda of executives, payers, and consumers, competing priorities, such as financial sustainability, patient engagement, regulatory standards, and governmental demands, remain organizational priorities. Nursing represents the largest health care profession in the United States and has the ability to influence the culture of patient safety and quality. It is essential for hospital leadership to provide a culture whereby nurses and staff are actively engaged and feel comfortable speaking up. Transparency is critical in the strategy and implementation of improving quality and safety.

This article describes important aspects of health-care quality, quality improvement (QI), patient safety (PS), and approaches to research on QI/PS efforts. Common terminology to facilitate an understanding of QI and PS research is reviewed. Models for understanding system and process performance are discussed. Introductory considerations to QI data and QI research analytical considerations are provided.

Emerging changes in the United States' healthcare delivery model have led to renewed interest in data-driven methods for managing quality of care. Analytics (Data plus Information) plays a key role in predictive risk assessment, clinical decision support, and various patient throughput measures. This article reviews the application of a pediatric risk score, which is integrated into our hospital's electronic medical record, and provides an early warning sign for clinical deterioration. Dashboards that are a part of disease management systems, are a vital tool in peer benchmarking, and can help in reducing unnecessary variations in care.

This article examines the current role of telehealth as a tool in the delivery of pediatric health care. It defines telemedicine and telehealth and provides an overview of different types of telehealth services. The article then explores the potential of telehealth to improve pediatric health care quality and safety through increased access to care, enhanced communication, expanded educational opportunities, and better resource utilization. It also discusses current challenges to the implementation of telehealth, including technological, financial, and licensing barriers, as well as provider, patient, and legal concerns.

PEDIATRIC CLINICS OF NORTH AMERICA

THE CLINICS ARE AVAILABLE ONLINE!
Access your subscription at:
www.theclinics.com

Foreword

Pediatric Safety, Quality, and Informatics

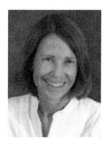

Bonita F. Stanton, MD
Consulting Editor

Of the "new frontiers" in medicine over the past few decades, arguably none has been as dramatic as "patient safety in the clinical setting." For decades, physicians and hospital personnel had assumed that hospital staff either (or both) were doing all that could be done or were achieving a high level of safe care for their patients. The release in 1999 of the withering report, *To Err Is Human: Building a Safer Health System*, by the Institute of Medicine (IOM) clearly and unequivocally exploded that myth. Among the countless attention-generating facts revealed in the report was the estimate of 44,000 to 98,000 deaths annually in the United States due to preventable medical errors. This report and a rapidly growing awareness of the problem led in 2005 to the passage of the Patient Safety and Quality Improvement Act and countless other federal, state, local, and health systems–based systems and approaches to decreasing medical errors.

The timing of the IOM report was important. The advent of electronic computerized systems, including the electronic medical record, has facilitated data-gathering and tracking and the development and deployment of safety checks. Medical education curricula for physicians, nurses, pharmacists, technicians, and the rest of the hospital staff explicitly address patient safety in both primary education and annual retraining efforts. Adverse events are now tracked—publicly—with the explicit expectation that the entire medical staff aggressively participate in achieving the established goals. This is a topic of great importance to all health care providers—and patients—and clearly is of great interest. PubMed contains 10,189 articles published in the past five years that address the topic of "patient safety in health care."

In this fascinating issue of *Pediatric Clinics of North America*, Dr Srinivasan Suresh and his colleagues provide clear and compelling descriptions of the many tools and approaches available to pediatricians regarding patient safety and report are what

Pediatr Clin N Am 63 (2016) xv–xvi
http://dx.doi.org/10.1016/j.pcl.2016.01.002
0031-3955/16/$ – see front matter © 2016 Published by Elsevier Inc.

pediatric.theclinics.com

hospital systems are doing to make the health care delivery systems safer places for your patients!

Bonita F. Stanton, MD
School of Medicine
Wayne State University
1261 Scott Hall
540 East Canfield, Suite 1261
Detroit, MI 48201, USA

E-mail address:
bstanton@med.wayne.edu

Preface

The Intersection of Safety, Quality, and Informatics: Solving Problems in Pediatrics

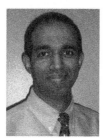

Srinivasan Suresh, MD, MBA, FAAP
Editor

Providing safe and high-quality care to infants and children is always a key priority for pediatricians and health care organizations. Although "safety" has been one of the domains of health care quality,[1] thousands of medical errors caused by the health care system itself continue to occur. Over the past few years, information technology has come to the forefront not only to improve disease specific outcomes, but also to facilitate the measurement and implementation of safe and high-quality care. Focused research in children has shown that problems and solutions in pediatric safety and quality have several unique aspects. The science of informatics (data plus meaning), as it relates to pediatrics, has to target population health and simultaneously address the rising costs associated with implementation and maintenance of computerized systems for care coordination, while at the same time contribute toward excellence in patient care. The tools available to measure, standardize, and peer-benchmark safety and quality metrics need to be refined as we drive toward the "triple aim" (better health, better health care at lower cost).[2]

Some of the exciting areas that fall under the intersection of pediatric safety, quality, and informatics are the application of big data and predictive analytics, addressing barriers to wider usage of clinical pathways, harnessing the power of medical device technologies, and the growing role of telemedicine. There should be continued emphasis in educating pediatric residents and fellows on the principles of pediatric quality and safety. The modern electronic medical record has become an indispensable component of clinical research.

Given the reach and readership of *Pediatric Clinics of North America*, this issue on "Quality of Care and Information Technology" strives to address the above areas as well as analyze current challenges in the realm of pediatric safety, quality, and informatics. The authors, who are experts in various pediatric care settings (hospital

Pediatr Clin N Am 63 (2016) xvii–xviii
http://dx.doi.org/10.1016/j.pcl.2016.01.001
0031-3955/16/$ – see front matter © 2016 Published by Elsevier Inc.

medicine, intensive care, emergency medicine, clinical informatics, nursing, and quality improvement research), provide an overview to widen the knowledge base of the practicing pediatrician and help them apply the content of these articles to their everyday practice.

Srinivasan Suresh, MD, MBA, FAAP
Children's Hospital of Pittsburgh of UPMC
University of Pittsburgh School of Medicine
Pittsburgh PA, USA
suresh@chp.edu

REFERENCES

1. Institute of Medicine (IOM). Crossing the Quality Chasm: A New Health System for the 21st Century. Washington, DC: National Academy Press; 2001.
2. Berwick DM, Nolan TW, Whittington J. The triple aim: care, health, and cost. Health Aff 2008;27(3):759–69.

Population Health and Pediatric Informatics

Emily C. Webber, MD

KEYWORDS

- Population health • Health information technology • Meaningful use
- Health disparities

KEY POINTS

- Pediatric clinical care incorporates many of the social determinants of health into clinical practice; this alignment positions pediatricians to help address many health disparities.
- Health information technology and electronic medical records (EMRs) use by pediatricians support medical care delivery; other areas of population health require growth in the types of data and application of informatics.
- Clinical informatics can address health disparities by promoting EMR features that support population health, development of population health information systems, and semantic health information exchange.

INTRODUCTION

Over the last decade, electronic medical records (EMRs) have been implemented and studied at an unprecedented rate, providing increased collections of longitudinal clinical data as well as automated reporting. There has also been increasing engagement of patients in accessing their own health data, and a fundamental shift in the stewardship and use of that health data. However, a great section of pediatric patients and pediatricians remain underserved in their exposure to some of the most promising aspects of technology for this purpose—that of the impact on population health.

Large amounts of data pertinent to population health are generated outside of medical care venues but are not yet systematically incorporated into patient decision-making. True semantic interoperability that allows for relevant data exchange is still in its infancy. Hospitals and health systems struggle to balance limited resources for maintaining necessary security and operations of their EMR systems, while providers and patients await the promise of patient-specific plans and data that will help realize the full potential of "going digital." Health systems and physicians are reaching outside of traditional health care venues to develop strategic efforts to address population health—either in how it is assessed and measured or how it will be impacted by their efforts.

Conflict of Interest: Dr E.C. Webber has identified no professional or financial affiliations for herself or her spouse.
Department of Pediatrics, Indiana University School of Medicine, Riley Hospital at IU Health, 705 Riley Hospital Drive, Room 3008, Indianapolis, IN 46202, USA
E-mail address: ewebber@iuhealth.org

In this article, the tenets of population health are explored, including the digital divide, how population health aligns with pediatric practice, successful applications of technology to pediatric population health issues, and the challenges that must be overcome for pediatricians and their patients to benefit from technology.

WHAT IS POPULATION HEALTH?

Modern models of population health have become widespread in the last decade, defined in 2003 by Kindig and Stoddart[1] as "the health outcomes of a group of individuals, including the distribution of such outcomes within the group." Determinants of population health outcomes include medical care, individual behavior, social environment, physician environment, and genetics. Although the delivery of medical care consumes the most resources, successful public health interventions target the determinants that can be changed and reduce inequalities between populations. By reducing health disparities and inequities among different groups of people, the negative impact of the social determinants can be controlled and mitigated and the greatest impact on outcomes realized.

The World Health Organization (WHO) reported in 2008 that social determinants of health were the main cause of health inequities in all countries and were responsible for the most diseases and injuries.[2] This finding is particularly poignant in the United States, where many resources are dedicated to delivery of medical care rather than improvements that may provide population health benefits.[3]

Population health aims to improve the health of the entire population, and the definition of health expands to accommodate this idea. Many population health policies approach a broad definition of health put forth by the WHO in 1946 as "a state of complete physical, mental, and social well-being and not merely the absence of disease or infirmity."[4] Thus, many consider the population health composed of outcomes, patterns of health determinants, and the interventions that link the two (**Fig. 1**).

One of the most prominent examples of a public health awareness campaigns is the Healthy People 2020 outreach project.[5] Launched in December 2010, the project outlined a decade-long plan to improve the health of all American citizens. Healthy People has worked since the 1980s on community collaborations, informed health decision, and the impact of prevention.

Healthy People identifies approximately 1200 objectives divided into 40 public health topic areas. The project also identifies a set of leading health indictors as social determinants of health and divides them into 12 topics, seen in **Box 1**. Among the lead federal agencies partnering with Healthy People is the Office of the National Coordinator for Health Information Technology. As of March 2014, many of the leading health indicators were listed as "target met" (15.4%) or "improving" (38.5%). Many of the population health determinants align closely with elements of standard pediatric care.[6]

THE DIGITAL DIVIDE

The social determinants of health are also broadly impacted by access to Internet and other digital tools, sometimes called the "digital divide." Access to the Internet aligns with other disparities and relates to determinants of health in a balance. For example, access to Internet can increase access to medical care, but is related to one's physical and social environment. The Pew Internet Project first assessed this disparity in 2000 and provided updated findings in 2012.[7] One in 5 American adults surveyed do not use the Internet. Those with a disability, less education, and lower household earnings were least likely to have Internet access. Senior citizens and those who spoke Spanish as a primary language were also less likely to have Internet access. Of note, the Pew

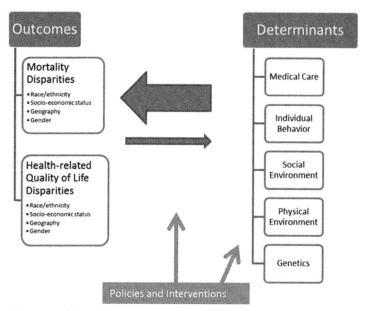

Fig. 1. Relationship of disparities to outcomes; social determinants of health greatly impact disparities. (*Courtesy of* David A Kindig MD, PhD, Madison, WI.)

study also illustrated an increase in the use of mobile devices to access Internet services overall. Eighty-eight percent of American adults have a cell phone, and other Internet-capable mobile devices are also growing.[7] Health care organizations in particular are beginning to use mobile strategies to reach undeserved groups and narrow the gap in Internet accessibility.[8]

Although health information technology (IT) can improve information and even access to promote equity, it cannot reverse deep rooted disparities that lead to gaps in health and health services.[9] Current health IT is well suited to identifying these inequities and informing possible solutions, particularly in the use of EMRs.[10] Indeed, the largest investment of applying technology to population health concerns remains EMRs. As EMR development continues, there has also been rapid development of innovative health-related applications of health IT.

These applications, including applications on mobile devices, 3-dimensional printers for prosthetics and complex surgery planning, and social media to connect communities and support initiatives, must become an adjunct to EMR uses to improve health. EMRs impact the delivery of medical care, but cannot address all the social determinants of health. Data arising from sources external of the medical care delivery

Box 1
Healthy people social determinants of health: leading health indicators

Access to health services	Nutrition, physical activity, and obesity
Clinical preventive services	Oral health
Environmental quality	Reproductive and sexual health
Injury and violence	Social determinants
Maternal, infant, and child health	Substance abuse
Mental health	Tobacco

venues will be key in the success of population health information models and EMR population health solutions.

ALIGNMENT OF PEDIATRIC PRACTICE WITH POPULATION HEALTH

The practices, procedures, institutions, and disciplines required to achieve population health are tied closely to essential elements of pediatric practice.[11] This alignment can be described in 4 key examples: the value pediatric places on social determinants of health, the practice of the well child examination, correlation of pediatric preventative care on adult health outcomes, and extension of care into non-health care venues.

First, pediatrics has a large body of research supporting the concept of social determinants as related to child health and adulthood.[12] Although experts in the delivery of medical care, pediatricians have also incorporated interventions, advocacy, interventions, and education into their standard practice. Pediatric research identifies key points in development which have a disproportionately high impact on outcomes. These key points are particularly influential, temporary detailed social determinants of health. Children exposed to adverse living environments (such as violence, abuse, or parental depression) have an increased risk of cardiovascular disease, depression, and suicide.[13] In addition, a stressful living environment can increase the chances of adopting health-adverse behaviors (smoking and substance abuse).[14]

Pediatrics has also incorporated advocacy as a core value, which involves engaging communities and evaluating individual patient needs. This practice emerged as a critical part of clinical care because it reflects the reality of a child's life; it happens to correlate with many social and economic determinants of health as well.[9] For example, recommending a dietary change in order to combat the risk of obesity aligns with a clinical practice guideline; however, this recommendation will be less successful if made to a lower income family that does not have a grocery store or access to fresh produce in their neighborhood.

Second, a pediatric well child examination and history compass data elements about home life and community, which tend to be more extensive and nuanced that the history obtained from an adult patient. This finding is particularly evident in the high-risk assessment screening frequently used in adolescent patients, known as the HEADSS (high-risk assessment of adolescent) assessment.[15] Additional examples of data gathered as part of routine well child care aligns with population health determinants is seen in **Box 2**.

Third, a key portion of pediatric care remains the link between child and adult health outcomes. Anticipatory guidance places emphasis on developing autonomy and the deferred benefits of teaching coping skills and making choices to promote health. Healthy habits that start in childhood can directly correlate with adult wellness.

Finally, pediatric practice involves communicating with school settings and assessing community resources, particularly for education. This expansion of pediatric care beyond the traditional walls of a clinic or hospital not only increases the benefit to the nonsick population but also can shape the policies that drive funding and resources, so that "health" rather than "health care" (or "medical care") has a priority within public and population health priorities.[12]

HOW HAS PEDIATRIC CARE AND POPULATION HEALTH BEEN SUPPORTED BY HEALTH INFORMATION TECHNOLOGY?

Most of the examples of health IT impacting population health outcomes are rooted in the delivery of medical care. This is not due to lack of awareness of the need for comprehensive population health information models and records, but is more a reflection of the information one is able to glean from the implementation of EMRs as the most prevalent example of health IT. Even with widespread EMR adoption, gaps exist which shape the available examples of success.

Box 2		
Components of the well child visit and correlation with population health determinants		
Well Child Care Assessment	**Topics Addressed**	**Population Health Determinant**
Preventative care	Vaccination	Medical care
Social history	School performance	Education
Social history	Living environment	Physical environment
HEADSS	Home safety	Physical environment
HEADSS	School performance, goals, and attitude	Education, social environment, and individual behavior
HEADSS	Activity, physical exercise, employment	Individual behaviors
HEADSS	Drug use	Social environment, individual behavior
HEADSS	Sexuality, sexual activity, history of pregnancy or sexually transmitted diseases	Social environment, individual behavior
HEADSS	Mental health	Social environment, individual behavior
Nutrition	Diet	Local food systems and agriculture; social environment
Developmental screening	Early childhood development	Medical care

In a survey administered in 2012,[16] a majority (79%) of pediatricians who responded indicated they were using an EMR, indicating a significant increase from the previous survey 5 years before. However, only 31% had basic functionally, and only 14% had a fully functional EMR. Even within EMR adoption, disparities exist. Providers seeing a high number of public insurance patients were more likely to use an EMR, most likely because of their eligibility for meaningful use (MU) of financial incentives; smaller practices (solo or 2 physician) were least likely to adopt an EMR at this point in time.

The survey of ambulatory pediatricians reflects an overall lower adoption rate and adoption of basic instead of full functionality, which can also be seen in national data from the Office of the National Coordinator (ONC). **Fig. 2** illustrates office-based physicians that attested successfully to MU; the distribution is heterogeneous, ranging from no physicians in geographically remote areas to high adoption scattered throughout the country. In contrast, **Fig. 3** illustrates hospital adoption, which is nearly uniform nationally.

Despite the implementation gap in EMR adoption between hospitals and office-based physicians, health IT in general has great potential in reducing disparities, facilitating behavior changes, and improving health care. With time, this should inform and enrich public health efforts, thereby enhancing health outcomes.[17] In a brief report in 2010, the ONC outlined how health IT might address current disparities and particularly address needs in underserved communities (**Table 1**).

The applications of health IT to pediatric population health are wide and varied, in both their impact and their reproducibility. Although a comprehensive review is beyond the scope of this article, there are some examples that illustrate both the catalyst of the Health Information Technology for Economic and Clinical Health (HITECH) and MU financial investment and the applicability to underserved populations. These examples can be grouped as follows:

I. EMR use and clinical decision support tools for population health outcomes
II. Consumer e-health tools
III. Population health information systems
IV. Health information exchange (HIE)

Telemedicine and telehealth should also be considered in this group and is addressed elsewhere.

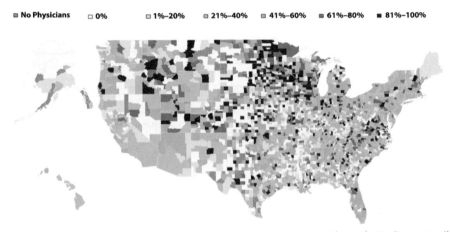

Fig. 2. Distribution of office-based physicians demonstrating MU through Medicare, April 2015. Note: Ambulatory Medical doctors and doctors of osteopathy only. (*From* Office of the National Coordinator for Health Information Technology. Office-based Physicians that have Demonstrated Meaningful Use through the Medicare EHR Incentive Program, Health IT Dashboard. http://dashboard.healthit.gov/dashboards/physicians-medicare-meaningful-use.php. July 2015.)

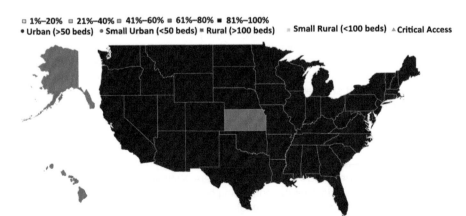

Fig. 3. Percentage of Medicare-eligible hospitals demonstrating MU, April 2015. Note: Hospitals eligible to participate in Medicate EHR Incentive Program only. (*From* Office of the National Coordinator for Health Information Technology. Hospitals that have Demonstrated Meaningful Use through the Medicare EHR Incentive Program, Health IT Dashboard. http://dashboard.healthit.gov/dashboards/hospitals-medicare-meaningful-use.php. July 2015.)

Table 1
Understanding the impact of health information technology in underserved communities and those with health disparities

	Current Disparities	Potential Impact of Health IT
Quality of care	Disparities exist for underserved populations for measures of quality that include effectiveness, patient safety, and timeliness.	Health IT tools can improve providers' decision-making processes as it relates to the needs of special populations, facilitate quality improvement reporting, and increase access to a broader range of quality health care services.
Access to care	Disparities exist in health insurance coverage, patient perceptions of need, and potentially avoidable hospital admissions.	Health IT including telehealth and distance medicine can improve access to specialist services and ancillary services, such as case management, transportation, and translation and can assist in providing free or low-cost preventative health services.
Health outcomes	Underserved populations are more likely to experience health outcome disparities, which vary from differences in morbidity and mortality rates for cancer and other illnesses to other measures of health.	The impact of health IT on health care delivery, safety, and patient engagement has the potential to improve health outcomes for the underserved.
Patient engagement	Lack of patient involvement in their own care can impact health, resulting in less preventive care and poorer understanding of their conditions and care, among other impacts. Lack of involvement may be due to lack of cultural sensitivity on the part of providers, health literacy on the part of patients, or a general feeling that it is not the patient's prerogative or responsibility to take an active role.	Health IT can aid in educating users about their condition and their treatment options as well as improve health literacy in general. Health IT can also help aid providers in offering more targeted care that addresses the cultural and language needs of their patients and that encourages patients to stay actively involved in their own health care plan.
Chronic disease management	Data have shown that underserved populations are more likely to exhibit signs of poor management of chronic disease, such as higher rates of hospital admissions for short-term complications associated with chronic diseases.	Health IT tools can facilitate improved coordination of care for individuals with chronic diseases, and consumer-oriented health IT tools can promote more active patient involvement, resulting in better management of chronic disease.

From NORC. Case Study 10 from the Office of the National Coordinator. 2010. Available at: https://www.healthit.gov/sites/default/files/pdf/hit-underserved-communities-health-disparities.pdf. Accessed September 1, 2015.

Electronic Medical Records and Clinical Decision Support

EMRs have been the most obvious investment in technology that directly impacts medical care. The HITECH act as part of American Recovery and Reinvestment Act in 2009 was a groundbreaking investment of public funds in the United States to drive adoption of certified EMRs. Although the clinical informatics community does not have full consensus regarding what constitutes consequential and significant application of an EMR to patient care, the MU criteria that define whether a hospital or provider is using the EMR have changed the landscape of both implementation and use.

Although only a few functions are categorized as public health initiatives under MU, there is immense potential for the application of MU criteria to impact social determinants. The widespread adoption of EMRs under MU, as well as reports of successful application of clinical decision support, should both be considered in this impact.

Meaningful use criteria for public health

HIPPA (Health Insurance Portability and Accountability Act) of 1996 evolved to include governance of sharing health data as well as breach and security rules. It does allow for sharing of medical data, and more recently EMR data, for specific health purposes. The HITECH act as noted above brought significant funding (more than $28 billion since enactment) for those physicians and hospitals using EMRs, along with granular, specific operational certification rules. These rules became known as the MU criteria.

MU is defined as the use of certified electronic health record (EHR) technology to achieve 4 main goals, 3 of which are directly related to population health:

1. Improve quality, safety, efficiency, and reduce health disparities
2. Engage patients and family
3. Improve care coordination, and population and public health
4. Maintain privacy and security of health information.[18]

Attestation to MU by a provider or hospital is directly tied to the Centers for Medicare and Medicaid (CMS) Incentive Program, and objectives were rapidly identified and adopted in 3 stages (**Table 2**).[19] Earlier participants, who began attesting to their use in 2011, were able to receive the maximum financial incentives. Conversely, providers and hospitals who do not attest will begin receiving penalties from CMS in 2015.

Although not formally identified as a high-level objective until stage 3, certified EHR technology is required to perform, and MU has required attestation for, 3 functions most like to support public health and population–based programs[18]:

- Interfacing with immunization registries to transmit electronic data as directed by public health agencies;
- Electronically recording, modifying, retrieving, and submitting syndromic surveillance data;
- Electronically recording, modifying, retrieving, and submitting reportable clinical laboratory results using Health Level Seven standards.

Clinical decision support in pediatrics

Assessment and integration of clinical guidelines; prioritizing social determinants of health The manner in which pediatricians and pediatric practices gather data and information about maternal health and wellness is an enormous opportunity. Identifying the sectors that are known to improve health outcomes can align a health care effort with a higher impact on the overall population health as well. This early identification, and integration of technology, particularly into the EMR itself, can both broaden the scope and increase the chances of success.

Table 2
Summary of meaningful use stages

Stage 1 (2011–2012): Data Capture and Sharing	Stage 2 (2014): Advance Clinical Processes	Stage 3 (2016): Improved Outcomes
Electronically capturing health information in a standardized format	More rigorous HIE	Improving quality, safety, and efficiency, leading to improved health outcomes
Using that information to track key clinical conditions	Increased requirements for e-prescribing and incorporating laboratory results	Decision support for national high-priority conditions
Communicating that information for care coordination processes	Electronic transmission of patient care summaries across multiple settings	Patient access to self-management tools
Initiating the reporting of clinical quality measures and public health information	More patient-controlled data	Access to comprehensive patient data through patient-centered HIE
Using information to engage patients and their families in their care		Improving population health

The continued challenge of presenting the right information at the right time on the right patient is a constant struggle. Prioritizing the clinically relevant information requires expertise in both clinical practice and informatics. Effective integration of recommendations into EMRs impacts the quality of the data that is provided to the clinician and the patient as well as any attestations to registries or external databases. Finnell and colleagues[20] addressed the Bright Futures collection of preventative pediatric guidelines using guideline implementability appraisal v 2.0. Bright Futures, published by the American Academy of Pediatrics, contains 2161 action items. The investigators consolidated these into 245 recommendations and identified 21% (n = 52) that were actionable. Nearly all the recommendations addressed screening. A minority (n = 13) addressed anticipatory guidance.

This type of coordination should help inform EMR design so that the highest priority items are integrated. The methodology researchers used to make that prioritization could be used to adopt recommendations for EMR integration. Determining whether a guideline is actionable should be a consideration in its overall value.[21] Population health and the social determinants of health are often criticized for being too broad; this type of analysis could help in modeling the broad needs of population health information systems as well as in EMR aiding in the delivery of medical care.

Use of the electronic medical records demographic features to predict and provide medical care A great deal of patient demographic information is documented in EMR; however, there are few examples using that data to link to other information, which could provide important context for the care provided. One example is described by researchers who were able to correlate admission and demographic data from their EMR with that obtained by the US Census.[22] Researchers were able link patients to their census tract and found a higher number of admissions (up to 6-fold more) for both bronchiolitis and pneumonia occurring within lower socioeconomic tracts of the country. They also found that poverty and the quality of the housing were strongly correlated with a return visit to the hospital. This type of research, using data about the social determinants of health in a community, can help target community and outreach resources where they are needed most. In addition, incorporating data about the social and physical environment provides a more comprehensive picture for the medical team.

Another powerful example of informatics and health IT powering population health involves tying individual patient information to larger groups of data to build immediately applicable predictive models. This example was recently described in a collaboration between MultiCare Health System and the University of Washington.[23] Data scientists used large amounts of data to create a model to predict which patients were at high risk for readmission. Through the use of a cloud platform (Microsoft's Azure), researchers were able to scale their efforts to match the volume of data.[24] Patients' case reports, even when incomplete, were able to be compared with those of thousands of other patients and take into account their unique social determinants. This "big data" element was coupled with an innovative engagement strategy—to show the patients themselves the readmission risk, to help provide suggestions for treatments, and to inform the ultimate choices.

Electronic Health Tools for Consumers

Population health features of large commercial EMRs are still early in development,[25] and initiatives as previously described are usually produced at large academic centers with the ability to adapt vendor EMRs and/or build custom tools. As a result, much consumer innovation occurs outside of the EMR. These applications that could contribute data to understanding nonmedical care determinants are guided by financial pressures of the health care industry as consumer need.

One such project is the "Text4baby" initiative undertaken by Whittaker and colleagues.[26] The project established the first free nationwide text message service. Working with established medical groups to set the content, the project eventually reached more than 100,000 women, many in lower income areas where access to health care would have been limited. Most participated in the prenatal period, receiving the 117 messages (sample messages in **Box 3**); however, around 75% of enrollees continued receiving messages through their infants first year of life.

Box 3
Sample messages from the "Text4baby" initiative

Free msg: Congratulations, you're going to be a mom! Text4baby wishes you a happy and healthy pregnancy. Thanks for including us in this special time.

Free msg: You can choose who you see for pregnancy care. Midwives, family docs, OBs & nurse practitioners can all provide care. Call 800-311-2229 for free/low-cost care & to find a provider who's right for you.

Free msg: The flu can be dangerous for pregnant women & their babies. Talk to your doctor about seasonal flu & H1N1 flu shots. More from CDC: 1-800-232-4636.

Free msg: Get your baby off to a great start! You can help your baby's development by taking a prenatal vitamin each day. It should have 600 mcg of folic acid.

Free msg: For a healthy baby, visit a doctor or midwife early & keep all of your appointments. Hear your baby's heartbeat. See how fast she grows!

Free msg: Give your baby a good start by not drinking alcohol, smoking, or using drugs. For help, call 800-784-8669 (smoking); 800-662-4357 (drugs & alcohol).

From Whittaker R, Matoff-Stepp S, Meehan J, et al. Text4baby: development and implementation of a national text messaging health information service. Am J Public Health 2012;102(12):2207–13; with permission.

The project used mobile technology in order to improve accessibility to health information for a population of pregnant women who otherwise may have had a lack of access to such regular, reliable, and informed advice. Currently, most examples of these consumer tools are not yet able to integrate easily into EMR for use in physician decision making. However, they do create sets of data that population health scientists, as well as public health advocates, can use to target specific populations.

Population Health Information Systems

All determinants of public health can be impacted by technology; however, as previously mentioned most resources and research have focused on the delivery of medical care in the treatment of disease. As health systems have shifted to focus on prevention as well as treatment and management of disease, health IT has begun a necessary evolution to manage, reconcile, secure, and interpret wider and more diverse data sources.

The need for a robust population health record in the United States has been described by multiple groups since the 1990s.[27–29] The International Organization for Standardization stated a population health record would include "aggregated and usually deidentified data. It may be obtained directly from EHRs or created de novo from other electronic repositories. It is used for public health and other epidemiological purposes, research, health statistics, policy development, and health services management."[29]

In a commentary from 2010, Friedman and Parrish[30] proposed a population health strategy or information model, which should include the purposes, uses, and content details in **Table 3**.

Table 3	
Proposed structure for population health information system	
Purpose	Document the state of and influences on the health of a defined population
Uses	• Monitoring population health status and outcomes • Conducting community health assessments and health impact assessments • Identifying population health disparities • Designing public health interventions, programs, and policies • Targeting interventions and programs to specific populations • Evaluating the impacts and outcomes of interventions, programs, and policies • Supplying feedback to providers of information • Supporting public health and health care personnel
Primary intended users	Health departments, community-based organizations with responsibilities for public health, public health clinics and practitioners, and some health care providers
Content	Aggregated data, such as statistics, measures, and indicators (mostly quantitative, but some might be ordinal or nominal, ie, the presence or absence or extent of enforcement of a particular policy)
Data sources	• Ongoing population surveys • Vital registration • Public health surveillance • Environmental sampling • Medicare and other payer claims • Population censuses • Public health practice–related programs • State-based hospital discharge

Adapted from Friedman DJ, Parrish RG. The population health record: concepts, definition, design, and implementation. J Am Med Inform Assoc 2010;17:359–66; with permission.

The investigators noted the data necessary to make additional progress are contained in silos of data that do not communicate effectively. They suggested that a successful electronic population health record would need to be based on a population health framework and be more inclusive in the factors influencing health. This idea is in contrast to the traditional focus of EMRs on the delivery of medical care.

Although there is not an example of a comprehensive population health information model embedded in a single EMR or geographic setting, both health information exchanges (HIE) and databases of population health information are examples of parts of EMRs serving an integral purpose in population health.

1. *HIE as a population health tool.* Several examples in the literature describe rapid data collection and exchange of individual patients, or aggregating data for patients from several sources (hospitals, laboratories, and other clinics) for exchange with health departments and organizations like the Centers for Disease Control and Prevention (CDC).[31–33] The use of HIE is still evolving, and inclusion in MU has served as a great catalyst; however, research reflects a small group of providers, and this type of functionality is not widespread in use.

2. *Databases for population health and web-based data query.* An electronic registry is one example of a population health information system. The CDC, the National Cancer Registry, and state health departments may curate collections of data for population health purposes. Some of these groups allow for customized queries of one or more population-based data sets, known as a "Web-based data query system" (WDQS). This type of query can be helpful, especially in the absence of any other data source, even if most WDQS do not explicitly reflect a larger population health information strategy in their design.[34] However, electronic registries to help address disparities, because they allow for the inclusion of standardized data about race and ethnicity, can empower providers to provide culturally appropriate care.[35]

Health Information Exchange

The ability to exchange clinical data as well as other pieces of health information remains central to population health information models. HIE is defined by the National Alliance for Health information Technology as "the transfer of electronic health information such as laboratory results, clinical summaries, and medication lists among organizations according to nationally recognized standards."[36] A survey of ambulatory providers showed that in 2013 approximately two-thirds of US hospitals and nearly half of physician practices were engaged in some type of HIE with outside organizations.[37] This finding represents a sharp increase in the adoption of HIE from 2008, when HIE participation among hospitals was 41% and among physicians was about 17%.[38]

A literature review in Health Affairs evaluated the impact of HIE and found a lack of compelling evidence in the current literature supporting HIE for this purpose.[39] However, the review process was encouraging in how it was able to examine HIE with regard to aspects of public and population health, instead of focusing solely on the delivery of medical care. For example, the investigators grouped outcomes in the studies they reviewed by outcomes in the following categories:

- Disease surveillance (for example, automatic reporting of diseases requiring public health notification)
- Coordination of care (for example, communication between a patient's different providers)

- Health care use (for example, hospital or emergency department [ED] readmissions, redundant laboratory tests)
- Health care costs (for example, outcomes measured in dollars)
- Patient experience (for example, patient satisfaction)
- Quality-of-care measure (for example, hemoglobin A1c levels or medication adherence)

Ninety-four studies were analyzed: 74.1% were published after 2009 and only 2.1% were focused on disease surveillance. However, both studies looking at the use of HIEs for disease surveillance found a positive impact. The biggest finding was the lack of evidence in the literature drawing a clear line from HIE to benefit—either to patients directly or to other determinants of population health. The fact that several seminal studies around HIE are based on work done with a unique, mature, and robust HIE also demonstrates that HIE is extremely early in its applications. Most studies at this point are focused on whether the exchange took place, which makes sense given the functionality commanded by current legislation and most health systems abilities. The investigators recommended that "future studies should focus on settings other than adult hospitals and EDs such as primary care, public health, pediatric inpatient, and long-term care settings."

One of the more mature HIEs that produced some of the reviewed work is the Indiana Network for Patient Care (INPC), which was created by the Regenstrief Institute Center for Biomedical Informatics, handles about half a million secure transactions daily. This data include medical histories, laboratory test results, medication records, and treatment reports. Hospitals and providers can then access data from the contributing providers and health care settings in a standardized format using an application for EMR-like access (CareWeb) and data sharing (DOCS4DOCS).[40]

The INPC was launched in 1994 thanks to funding from the National Library of Medicine's initiative, established at a time before widespread EMR use, and achieved a critical mass early; this has allowed for new participants and functions with ease because competing HIEs are not a factor. Future HIE development will not have these conditions. Despite its size, the INPC exchange is limited to a small number of hospitals and providers it services compared with the national need for this type of accessibility. Far more physicians and patients will experience HIE that will be aligned and shaped by MU in the coming years.

CHALLENGES IN USING HEALTH IT TO PROMOTE POPULATION HEALTH

Application of the HITECH certified features of EHRs mandates the ability to support public health programs; however, there remain several barriers to success. Friedman and Parrish[30] speculate "Perhaps the most basic barrier to the population health records in the US is fragmentation of population health data collection and data stewardship responsibilities among federal, state, and local governments."

Fragmentation can be considered to have grown from several sources. These barriers can result from a lack of strategy and rapid growth, almost "naturally occurring" and certainly unintended in their evolution. The ONC released a National Roadmap to Interoperability, which described barriers to interoperability: lack of trust, misinterpretation and differences in privacy laws, aligning payment incentives, and insufficient standardization of health information.[41] Barriers can also arise out of deliberate actions, frequently from financial or competitive nature between health systems and EMRs. The motivation behind establishing these barriers could be argued to be "artificial," meaning their existence is not critical to the success or failure of the EMR system operation, but is present nonetheless.

A congressional report released in April 2015 delineates the differences between "organic" or intended barriers to interoperability, and the "artificial" barriers it defined as information blocking.[42] Examples are seen in **Box 4**. The report called information blocking the event in which "persons or entities knowingly and unreasonably interfere with the exchange or use of electronic health information." The report is a call for action, outlining a strategy to prevent restriction of health information by those with knowledge of the impact of their actions. The investigators recognize that "current economic incentives and characteristics of both health care and health IT markets create business incentives for some market participants to pursue and exercise control over information in ways that significantly limit its availability and use."

These 2 strategies together produce a hostile environment for interoperability and collaboration, leading to inertia in the population health EMR development. It makes it challenging to obtain permission to use data, standardize it, or collaborate on Web-based services. For example, exchange of information between vaccination registries would support timely clinical decision support, and therefore, effective administration of immunizations. However, both large vendor and custom EMR products have struggled to send and receive information between registries. Some states have more than registry, for example, In addition, although the vaccination schedule is published and revised each year with fairly consistent intervals, designing clinical decision support that applies conditional logic and reconciles vaccinations from multiple sources requires substantial resources and customization to achieve.

One additional element that contributes to the gap between clinical informatics potential and the reality of applied tools is a paucity of evidence as to the long-term benefits and efficacy of information exchange. Clinical informatics and population health—although not new ideas—are experiencing a new level of data exchange. Adapting to new tools and a much larger pool of data will take time, as will producing meaningful data and discourse on public health outcomes. The nature of population health outcomes assumes that the impact of changing a single health determinant may not be fully captured immediately, nor can it be predictably evaluated in isolation.

Clinical informatics as a discipline grew out during the last decade with a heavy focus on medical care. A large number of complex implementations and improvements of EMR in a relatively narrow time frame has produced most of the literature. As a result, measuring impact on patient care has been restricted thus far to reporting on successful process and short-term outcome measures (including finances).

Box 4
Examples of obstacles to health information exchange

Examples with unintended, "naturally occurring" features	Examples with deliberate, "artificial" features
Inconsistent adoption of health information standards	Technology (including EMRs) that requires substantial customization to exchange data
Lack of infrastructure to support data exchange	Heavy financial burdens for users of health IT that try to retrieve or share data
Security features	Deliberate design making it difficult to third party vendors
Need for data reconciliation when exchanged	Refusal of health systems to share patient data
Variation in state laws	
Examples with both unintended and deliberate features	
Variation in privacy laws	
Aligning payment incentives	

Population health outcomes, by contrast, are separated in time and space from the interventions.

FUTURE DIRECTIONS

In order for physicians and other health care leaders to realize the full potential of EMRs, the model of how a health system interacts with technology will need to adapt to include the measures of success as well as strategic goals. The continued challenge of improving and updating EMRs in large hospital-based settings remains; however, focus is shifting from purchase and implementation to information exchange and efficient information reconciliation. This shift allows for true semantic interoperability that enhances the medical care delivery. As financial viability for health care moves toward rewarding preventative care and long-term outcomes for chronic illnesses, instead of a fee-for-service model, this shift will also provide the data needed to shape the new metrics of success for health care system.

This shift will change the most widespread challenges to data capture in a diverse range of settings and will include traditional health care delivery environments such as ambulatory clinics. However, there will also be a need to both receive and reconcile data from health care delivery venues external to the health system, including clinics and hospitals, which may also be in competition with each other, as well as settings such as urgent care clinics and school clinics. In addition, data sources such as patients themselves, their mobile devices, and their medical equipment will need to be addressed.

Pediatric patients represent the early adopters of many forms of technology, and their parents and caregivers already use technology as an adjunct tool in managing health. Two elements of MU, E-prescribing and online access to patient records, are quickly becoming the expectation instead of the exception. Health IT outside of EMRs is also increasing—seeking additional education online, refilling a prescription using a pharmacy mobile application, or tracking activity using one of many health devices such as a personal mobile fitness device. Data sources from nonhospital, nonclinic venues represent information closely aligned with social determinants of health such as individual behaviors as well as the social and physical environment. Physicians and other health care leaders should anticipate that this new standard will continue to shape how technology is used and how EMRs are designed.

REFERENCES

1. Kindig D, Stoddart G. What is population health? Am J Public Health 2003;93(3): 380–3.
2. Meeting Report of World Conference of Social Determinants of Health held in Rio de Janeiro, Brazil. 2008. Available at: http://www.who.int/sdhconference/resources/Conference_Report.pdf. Accessed September 1, 2015.
3. McGinnis JM, Williams-Russo P, Knickman JR. The case for more active policy attention to health promotion. Health Aff 2002;21:78–93.
4. World Health Organization. WHO definition of Health, Preamble to the Constitution of the World Health Organization as adopted by the International Health Conference. New York, 19–22 June 1946. FP Grad. 2002. The Preamble of the Constitution of the World Health Organization. Bulletin of the World Health Organization. 80(12):982.
5. Healthy People 2020. Available at: http://www.healthypeople.gov/2020/default. Accessed September 1, 2015.

6. Healthy People 2020 indicators. Available at: http://www.healthypeople.gov/2020/leading-health-indicators/Healthy-People-2020-Leading-Health-Indicators%3A-Progress-Update. Accessed September 1, 2015.

7. Zickuhr K, Smith A. Digital differences. Washington, DC: Pew Charitable Trusts; 2012. Pew Internet and American Life Project. Available at: http://www.pewinternet.org/2012/04/13/digital-differences/. Accessed September 1, 2015.

8. Fox, Suzannah. Presentation: "The Power of Mobile". Available at: http://www.pewinternet.org/Commentary/2010/September/The-Power-of-Mobile.aspx. Accessed September 1, 2015.

9. Barclay G, Sabina A, Graham G. Population health and technology: placing people first. Am J Public Health 2014;104(12):2246–7.

10. Loonsk J. Minding the public's health IT. Government Health IT. Portland (ME): HIMSS Media; 2010. Available at: http://govhealthit.com/blog/minding-publics-health-it. Accessed September 1, 2015.

11. Friedman DJ, Parrish G, Ross DA. Electronic health records and US Public Health: current realities and future promise. Am J Public Health 2013;103(9):1560–7.

12. Corden TE, Kindig DA. Pediatric population health: determinants and policy paradigm. Pediatr Ann 2011;40(3):131–5.

13. Repetti RL, Taylor SE, Seeman TE. Risky families: family social environments and the mental and physical health of offspring. Psychol Bull 2002;128(2):330–66.

14. McEwen BS. Protective and damaging effects of stress mediators. N Engl J Med 1998;338(3):171–9.

15. Straub DM. Adolescent medicine. In: Siberry GK, Iannone R, editors. The Harriet Lane handbook. 15th edition. St Louis (MO): Mosby; 2000. p. 97.

16. Lehmann CU, O'Connor KG, Shorte VA, et al. Use of electronic health record systems by office-based pediatricians. Pediatrics 2015;135:e7.

17. Graham G. Using technology to improve minority health. Rockville (MD): Office of Minority Health; 2009. Available at: http://www.e-healthpolicy.org/docs/2009_Sessions/20090313_Dr%20Garth%20Graham_Hill_Briefing.pdf.

18. Definition of meaningful use. Available at: http://healthit.gov/providers-professionals/meaningful-use-definition-objectives. Accessed September 1, 2015.

19. Meaningful use objectives. Available at: http://healthit.gov/providers-professionals/meaningful-use-definition-objectives. Accessed September 1, 2015.

20. Finnell SM, Stanton JL, Downs SM. Actionable recommendations in the Bright Futures child health supervision guidelines. Appl Clin Inform 2014;5(3):651–9.

21. Biondich PG, Downs SM, Carroll AE, et al. Collaboration between the medical informatics community and guideline authors: fostering HIT standard development that matters. AMIA Annu Symp Proc 2006;36–40.

22. Beck AF, Florin TA, Campanella S, et al. Geographic variation in hospitalization for lower respiratory tract infections across one county. JAMA Pediatr 2015;169(9):846–54.

23. University of Washington news, "your heart is big data." Available at: https://www.tacoma.uw.edu/news/article/your-heart-big-data. Accessed September 1, 2015.

24. Dynamic hierarchical classification for patient risk-of-readmission, Senjuti Basu Roy, Ankur Teredesai, Kiyana Zolfaghar, Rui Liu, David Hazel, Stacey Newman, Albert Marinez, ACM KDD. 2015. Available at: http://cwds.uw.edu/dynamic-hierarchical-classification-patient-risk-readmission. Accessed September 1, 2015.

25. Cerner's HealtheIntent Platform. Available at: https://www.cerner.com/solutions/population_health/healthe_intent/. Accessed September 1, 2015.

26. Whittaker R, Matoff-Stepp S, Meehan J, et al. Text4baby: development and implementation of a national text messaging health information service. Am J Public Health 2012;102(12):2207–13.

27. American Medical Informatics Association, Board of Directors. A proposal to improve quality, increase efficiency, and expand access in the US health care system. J Am Med Inform Assoc 1997;4:340e1.

28. National Committee on Vital and Health Statistics. Assuring a health dimension for the national information infrastructure. Washington, DC: Department of Health and Human Services (US); 1998.

29. International Organization for Standardization. ISO/TR 20514: Health informatics electronic health record definition, scope, and context.

30. Friedman DJ, Parrish RG. The population health record: concepts, definition, design, and implementation. J Am Med Inform Assoc 2010;17:359–66.

31. Diamond CW, Mostashari F, Shirky C. Collecting and sharing data for population health: a new paradigm. Health Aff 2009;28:454–66.

32. Lazarus R, Yih K, Platt R. Distributed data processing for public health surveillance. BMC Public Health 2006;6:235.

33. McDonald CJ, Overhage JM, Barnes M, et al. The Indiana Network for Patient Care: a working local health information infrastructure. Health Aff 2005;24:1214–20.

34. Friedman DJ, Parrish RG. Characteristics and desired functionalities of state web-based data query systems. J Public Health Manag Pract 2006;12:119–29.

35. Engelberg Center for Health Care Reform at the Brookings Institution. How registries can help performance measurement improve care. 2010. Available at: http://www.rwjf.org/files/research/65448.pdf. Accessed September 1, 2015.

36. National Alliance for Health Information Technology. The National Alliance for Health Information Technology report to the Office of the National Coordinator for Health Information Technology on defining key health information technology terms [Internet]. Washington, DC: Department of Health and Human Services; 2008. Available at: http://www.nachc.com/client/Key%20HIT%20Terms%20Definitions%20Final_April_2008.pdf.

37. Hsiao CJ, Hing E. Use and characteristics of electronic health record systems among office-based physician practices: United States, 2001–2013. NCHS Data Brief 2014;(143):1–8.

38. Swain M, Charles D, Furukawa MF. Health information exchange among US non-federal acute care hospitals: 2008–2013. Washington, DC: Office of the National Coordinator for Health Information Technology; 2014. ONC Data Brief No. 17.

39. Rahukar S, Vest JR, Menachemi N. Despite the spread of health information exchange, there is little evidence on its impact on cost, use and quality of care. Health Aff 2015;34(3):477–83.

40. Indiana network for health information exchange. Available at: http://www.ihie.org/. Accessed September 1, 2015.

41. ONC, Connecting health and care for the nation: A shared nationwide interoperability roadmap draft version 1.0. 2015. Available at: http://www.healthit.gov/sites/default/files/nationwide-interoperability-roadmap-draft-version-1.0.pdf. Accessed September 1, 2015.

42. Report to Congress, April 2015. Report on Health Information Blocking. Available at: http://healthit.gov/sites/default/files/reports/info_blocking_040915.pdf. Accessed September 1, 2015.

Measurement, Standards, and Peer Benchmarking: One Hospital's Journey

Brian S. Martin, DMD, MHCDS

KEYWORDS

- Benchmarking • Pediatric • Solutions for Patient Safety
- Children's Hospital of Pittsburgh of UPMC

KEY POINTS

- Peer-to-peer benchmarking is an important component of rapid-cycle performance improvement in patient safety and quality-improvement efforts.
- Institutions should carefully examine critical success factors before engagement in peer-to-peer benchmarking in order to maximize growth and change opportunities.
- Solutions for Patient Safety has proven to be a high-yield engagement for Children's Hospital of Pittsburgh of University of Pittsburgh Medical Center, with measureable improvement in both organizational process and culture.

INTRODUCTION

Attention to quality, safety, and value in health care has undergone significant evolution over the past 25 years. Traditionally, patients, payers, and hospitals have approached the relationship from a relatively siloed perspective. More recently, efforts have been made to reframe the conversation toward a patient-centric, complex adaptive system. The adoption of the Affordable Care Act has served to accelerate this trend, including focus on patient safety, hospital-acquired conditions (HACs), and outcomes. These efforts have caused institutions to reevaluate what, when, and how they use metrics and analytics in order to improve health care delivery. Increasingly, leaders in health care are becoming fluent in quality management science, often referencing other industries for inspiration/guidance in the health care space. Many recognize the Donabedian framework of structure, process, and outcome, in conjunction with various process improvement tools (plan, do, study, act [PDSA], Lean) to drive organizational change efforts.

Externally, institutions face an evolving competitive landscape, with an increased appetite from patients, families, and insurers demanding data transparency on

Children's Hospital of Pittsburgh of UPMC, 7th Floor, Faculty Pavilion, 4401 Penn Avenue, Pittsburgh, PA 15224, USA
E-mail address: brian.martin@chp.edu

Pediatr Clin N Am 63 (2016) 239–249
http://dx.doi.org/10.1016/j.pcl.2015.11.004
0031-3955/16/$ – see front matter © 2016 Elsevier Inc. All rights reserved.

pediatric.theclinics.com

institutional performance. Health systems, payers, and patients find themselves increasingly aligned toward a goal of high-value (defined as outcomes/cost) health care. In addition to competitive market forces, payment incentives by the Centers for Medicare and Medicaid Services in the area of electronic health records (EHRs) and evolving regulatory standards from The Joint Commission (TJC) have provided a strong impetus for health systems to accelerate learning cultures and best-practice adoption.

This article begins with a brief review of the history of measurement, standards, and benchmarking, with a particular focus on pediatric-specific work led by the Agency on Healthcare Research and Quality (AHRQ). The author then discusses the success of the Ohio Collaborative (now known as Solutions for Patient Safety [SPS]), with remarks on critical success factors, including infrastructure in data/analytics and institutional cultural preparedness to ensure the highest yield from a benchmarking exercise.

Finally, the author uses the Children's Hospital of Pittsburgh of University of Pittsburgh Medical Center's (UPMC) (CHP) experience with SPS as a case study in peer-peer benchmarking, beginning with the history of the collaborative and the CHP's decision to participate. Furthermore, the author discusses the initial process of engagement and the effect of participation on the CHP's quality and safety process improvement efforts, people, and institutional culture.

HISTORY OF MEASUREMENT, STANDARDS, AND BENCHMARKING IN PEDIATRICS

For more than 20 years, the AHRQ of the US Department of Health and Human Services has been leading the charge for health care quality improvement and patient safety efforts. Beginning in the late 1990s, AHRQ-funded projects began to specifically focus on pediatric patients and processes related to patient safety.[1] Length of stay, hospital mortality, and increased hospital expenditures were the variables examined relative to their association to patient safety events.

In following suit to their adult counterparts, the development of quality indicators raises unique challenges in pediatric institutions. The AHRQ recognizes such considerations:

> These challenges include the need to carefully define indicators using administrative data, establish validity and reliability, detect bias and design appropriate risk adjustment, and overcome challenges of implementation and use. However, the special population of children invokes additional, special challenges. Four factors—differential epidemiology of child healthcare relative to adult healthcare, dependency, demographics, and development—can pervade all aspects of children's healthcare; simply applying adult indicators to younger age ranges is insufficient.[1]

Background on Pediatric Quality Indicators is provided in **Box 1**.

From the AHRQ, In conjunction with the AHRQ, the Child Health Corporatio of America (CHCA), the National Perinatal Information Center, and TJC serve to identify, define, and validate Pediatric Quality Indicators derived from hospital administrative data.[2] The current Pediatric Quality Indicators are noted in **Box 2**.

The AHRQ's work on pediatric-specific quality indicators (PQIs) served to provide a platform for institutions to benchmark against a valid, national standard. Beginning in 2012, the AHRQ began to provide benchmark data tables, enabling easier comparisons of nationwide comparative rates for the PQIs; data presented include observed rate and both numerator and denominator data for each indicator overall and stratified by sex, age group, and insurance status. An example of the overview benchmark data

---

Box 1
Background on AHRQ Pediatric Quality Indicators

Pediatric Quality Indicators

- Are used to help identify health care quality and safety problem areas in the hospital that need further investigation as well as for comparative public reporting, trending, and pay-for-performance initiatives

- Can provide a check on children's primary care access or outpatient services in a community by using patient data found in a typical hospital discharge abstract

- Apply to special characteristics of the pediatric population

- Include risk adjustment where appropriate

- Include *hospital-level* indicators to detect potential safety problems that occur during a patients hospital stay

- Include *area-level* indicators, which are conditions that may be prevented with good outpatient care

- Are publicly available without cost

- Can be downloaded at www.qualityindicators.ahrq.gov/pdi_download.htm

The Pediatric Quality Indicators are part of a set of software modules of the AHRQ's *Quality Indicators* developed by Battelle Memorial Institute, Stanford University, and the University of California, Davis under a contract with the AHRQ. The Pediatric Quality Indicators were released in 2006.

---

table for March 2015 is provided in **Table 1**, with greater detail in provider-level data table for neonatal iatrogenic pneumothorax in **Table 2**.

In summary, the AHRQ's work to provide standardization for national quality indicators serves as a foundation for institutions to benchmark their own performance against national goals to prevent avoidable patient safety events and improve health care delivery value to our nation's children. Other measurement tools, such as CHCA's Pediatric Health Information System can be used to augment and benchmark institutional performance.[3] In order to accelerate improvement efforts, interinstitutional communication regarding performance variation from the national benchmarks is critical to advance a culture of continuous quality improvement, engagement with data-driven decision making, and patient safety. From this need, the Ohio Collaborative was born.

SOLUTIONS FOR PATIENT SAFETY

Beginning in the 1980s, the Ohio Children's Hospital Association (OCHA) formed as a group of 6 children's hospitals to advocate for legislative, regulatory, and reimbursement issues. The association evolved to broaden its focus to include patient safety and quality efforts over the next 15 years. By 2005, it had launched a statewide effort to reduce preventable cardiac arrest outside the intensive-care-unit environment through the use of rapid-response teams. Following this success, a collaborative effort with member hospitals resulted in 5 pediatric quality and safety measures, which were adopted by the Ohio Department of Health. By 2009, OCHA extended to all pediatric centers in Ohio, forming the Ohio Children's Hospitals Solutions for Patient Safety (OCHSPS), now termed SPS.

Initial work of the OCHSPS focused on surgical site infections (SSIs) and adverse drug events (ADEs). These indicators, among others, are currently collectively

Box 2
Current AHRQ Pediatric Quality Indicators

The Pediatric Quality Indicators provide a perspective on potential complications and errors resulting from a hospital admission among children, adolescents, and, where specified, neonates.

Hospital-level indicators

- Accidental puncture or laceration
- Pressure ulcer
- Foreign body left in during procedure
- Central venous catheter–related bloodstream infections
- Iatrogenic pneumothorax in neonates
- Iatrogenic pneumothorax
- Neonatal mortality
- Bloodstream infections in neonates
- Pediatric heart surgery mortality
- Pediatric heart surgery volume
- Postoperative hemorrhage or hematoma
- Postoperative respiratory failure
- Postoperative sepsis
- Postoperative wound dehiscence
- Transfusion reactions

Area-level indicators (eg, county, state)

- Asthma admissions
- Diabetes short-term complications
- Gastroenteritis admissions
- Perforated appendix admissions
- Urinary tract infection admissions

considered HACs. Cardinal Health, a privately owned medical supply and pharmaceutical company, recognized the importance of OCHSPS's work and provided financial support.

Rapid-cycle process improvement efforts (PDSA) and training sessions were organized for the quality departments of member hospitals, along with data acquisition, transparency, and evolution of culture of safety. The end result was a decrease in SSIs by 60% and ADEs by 50% in approximately 1 calendar year.[4–9]

By 2011, Ohio children's hospitals had reduced serious safety events by 55% and serious harm events by 40%. Building on this success, by 2012, twenty-five children's hospitals joined the Ohio founding hospitals to form the Children's Hospitals' SPS. CHP initiated their collaboration as part of the first non-Ohio cohort.

GROUNDWORK FOR SUCCESS WITH SOLUTIONS FOR PATIENTS SAFETY

In early 2012, CHP was presented with the opportunity to participate in SPS. Senior leadership, including the president, chief medical officer, chief nursing officer, and senior

Table 1
March 2015 AHRQ benchmark data

Indicator	Label Provider-Level Indicators	Numerator	Denominator	Observed Rate per 1000 (=Observed Rate × 1000)
NQI #1	Neonatal iatrogenic pneumothorax rate	33	186,270	0.18
NQI #2	Neonatal mortality rate	6851	3,041,508	2.25
NQI #3	Neonatal blood stream infection rate	1596	63,379	25.18
PDI #1	Accidental puncture or laceration rate	1067	2,297,161	0.46
PDI #2	Pressure ulcer rate	62	226,690	0.27
PDI #3	Retained surgical item or unretrieved device fragment count	29	—	—
PDI #5	Iatrogenic pneumothorax rate	234	2,071,756	0.11
PDI #6	RACHS-1 pediatric heart surgery mortality rate	447	14,168	31.55
PDI #7	RACHS-1 pediatric heart surgery volume	16,857	—	—
PDI #8	Perioperative hemorrhage or hematoma rate	408	78,531	5.2
PDI #9	Postoperative respiratory failure rate	877	60,392	14.52
PDI #10	Postoperative sepsis rate	938	65,478	14.33
PDI #11	Postoperative wound dehiscence rate	48	42,923	1.12
PDI #12	Central venous catheter–related blood stream infection rate	1387	1,813,113	0.76
PDI #13	Transfusion reaction count	—	—	—
PSI #17	Birth trauma rate: injury to neonate	5636	2,974,363	1.89

Abbreviations: NQI, national quality indicator; PSI, patient safety indicator; PDI, pediatric quality indicator-provider level composite; RACHS, pediatric health surgery volume quality indicator.

Table 2
Provider-level indicators for neonatal iatrogenic pneumothorax

Indicator	Numerator	Denominator	Observed Rate per 1000 (= Observed Rate × 1000)
Overall	33	186,270	0.18
Females	14	92,876	0.15
Males	19	93,394	0.2
<1 y	33	186,270	0.18
Private	21	76,968	0.27
Medicare	—	578	—
Medicaid	—	96,621	—
Other	—	7122	—
Uninsured (self-pay/no charge)	—	4981	—

director of quality and safety, recognized the need to perform an audit of their ability to achieve the critical success factors necessary for maximum impact and engagement. The following areas were examined: infrastructure (data/analytics), organizational structure to effect change, tools for provider engagement, and organizational culture.

Infrastructure: Data

CHP began its journey toward a paperless hospital environment in 2003 with the adoption/implementation of the Cerner EHR platform. A strategy to reduce ADEs and medication safety was created in conjunction with installation of the EHR. To this end, computerized physician order entry (CPOE) combined with process retooling in CHP's pharmacy department was their first EHR-centric process improvement initiative. CPOE stands as the genesis point for our hospital's engagement with clinical informatics. Significant investments were made in provider, patient, and family education to create buy-in regarding the goals of transition from a paper-based record to EHR.[10] Over the next 9 years, CHP transitioned to full implementation of the Cerner platform in both outpatient and inpatient areas; by 2012, they achieved Stage 7 designation by Healthcare Information and Management Systems Society (HIMSS) Analytics, the highest level of clinical EHR utilization, as explained in **Fig. 1.**

CHP's foundation in clinical analytics and UPMC's significant investment in data warehouse infrastructure placed CHP in a position of strength regarding their ability to provide actionable data to the SPS collaborative.

Organizational Structure to Effect Change

The second critical success factor was CHP's ability to address the challenges and opportunities of a peer-to-peer benchmarking group. Platforms for engagement included shared leadership councils and workgroups in the nursing division, the Clinical Quality Oversight and Patient Safety Oversight Committee, Division Chiefs Committee, and the Medical Executive Committee.

CHP's recent MAGNET designation, noted to be the gold standard in nursing quality assessment, further encouraged their analysis that they had a system primed for success with nursing leaders who were receptive to productive change.[11] Their vision was that executive leadership, empowered with SPS data, would use these levers in order to accelerate the adoption of best practices developed and refined by the SPS engagement.

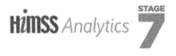

According to HIMSS Analytics, Stage 7 hospitals are considered to be completely paperless. In 2005, HIMSS launched the EMR Adoption Model to track adoption of EMR applications within hospitals and health systems. The EMRAM scores hospitals in the HIMSS Analytics Database on their progress in completing eight stages, with the goal of reaching Stage 7– the pinnacle of an environment where paper charts are no longer used to deliver patient care.

Stage 7 healthcare organizations support the sharing and use of patient data that ultimately improves process performance, quality of care and patient safety. Clinical information can be readily shared via standard electronic transactions, with all entities within health information exchange networks. This stage allows the healthcare organization to support the true sharing and use of health and wellness information by consumers and providers alike. Also at this stage, organizations use data warehousing and mining techniques to capture and analyze care data for performance improvement and advancing clinical decision support protocols.

Fig. 1. Description of HIMSS Stage 7. (*From* Agency for Healthcare Research and Quality, ahrq.gov.)

Finally, on engagement, CHP was prepared to develop an SPS leadership group, directed by the chief medical officer and coled by a nursing and physician leader. The interdisciplinary design would serve as the model for individual HAC teams, which would accordingly be coled by nursing and physician leaders who would be able to identify best practices and recruit frontline medical and nursing champions.

Tools for Provider Engagement with Benchmarking

The ability for physician, nursing, and administrative leaders to understand basic concepts of statistics and data analysis is critical for success in quality improvement.[12] To this end, CHP recognized the need for widespread education in statistical process control for frontline providers. The hospital engaged an expert in education in this discipline who provided sponsored education to hospital leaders/administration and medical and nursing staff. Education in this area challenges staff to deepen the context and understanding of CHP's performance relative to upper and lower control limits using statistical process control. This understanding, in conjunction with benchmarking data, enables focused, higher-yield interventions.

Institutional Culture

As evidenced by its early adopter status in CPOE, CHP is committed to innovation and continuous process improvement in their environment. CHP's parent organization, UPMC, is entirely supportive of this aspect of their mission. Congruent with their hospital efforts regarding patient- and family centered care, UPMC sponsors the Patient and Family Centered Care initiative (PFCC), which serves to promote a patient- and family centric culture within the institution.[13,14] Interdisciplinary, physician, nursing, and ancillary (patient support, dietary, environmental services) workgroups convene, collaborate, and innovate to provide a positive impact on the patient care experience.

A second UPMC system resource is the Donald Wolff Center for Innovation at UPMC. The Wolff Center exemplifies the movement from quality improvement (QI) expertise from a centralized function to an opportunity for dissemination of quality improvement expertise to frontline staff. To this end, resources, programming, and QI expertise provided by the Wolff Center serves as an additional positive force in driving CHP's institutional culture of improvement across CHP's staff. Resources, such as the PFCC and the Wolff Center, have primed CHP's institutional culture to create maximum impact from a benchmarking exercise.

RISK/BENEFIT FOR PARTICIPATING HOSPITALS

Participating in a national collaborative comes with both risk and reward. Organizations considering participation must be ready to provide specific, often sensitive information, including the use of quantitative data to support their claims. The contributions to a collaborative serve several purposes.

To understand where CHP stood within the pediatric community (their peers), they first determined what organizational processes were working and what processes had an opportunity for improvement. Ideally, peer-to-peer communication and best practice in processes and outcomes should be a continuous exercise. Determining these processes requires transparency both internally to and externally from their organization. Reflection on their own internal data dissemination processes lead CHP to retool both how often and in what format they provide data to their staff. This practice encourages organizational awareness, staff participation and professional growth, and a more cohesive work environment. Externally, their efforts as an organization will be visible to their peers for review.

Participation in this collaborative required a change in their organization's thinking. Adoption of a noncompetitive, collaborative posture toward patient safety requires a dose of humility and acceptance. A culture of intellectual honesty and willingness to challenge norms and face difficult decisions is critical in order to learn and improve. Risks of participation include correctly identifying areas of needed improvement, the potential of inaccurate metrics and event categorization, and the reality that there is much work to be done.

With the risks of participation come the benefits. Working collaboratively allows the opportunity to group think at a much greater level. Peers become valuable resources and assist in the guidance of process improvements. At any time, organizations are in various stages of similar processes. A national collaboration encourages and supports opportunities to review what ideas and implementations are effective and others that may need revision. What this yields is a highly refined, structured, and clear path to an end goal facilitated by the organization with support from others.[15] In order to grow as an organization, one must first admit and accept the need for help. Through the collaboration, CHP put aside competition and shared ideas collectively for the greater good of their patients.

CHILDREN'S HOSPITAL OF PITTSBURGH OF UNIVERSITY OF PITTSBURGH MEDICAL CENTER'S EXPERIENCE WITH SOLUTIONS FOR PATIENT SAFETY

Before engagement with SPS, CHP had performed groundwork on ADEs and ventilator-associated pneumonia care plans. However, during CHP's preengagement decision process, it was recognized that they also had significant institutional interest in hospital-acquired infections. Review of the current SPS benchmarking work also revealed areas of opportunity for CHP in additional HACs and patient safety events, including patient falls with injury and venous thrombolytic events. CHP was already taking action in many of these areas; however, participation in SPS challenged CHP to refine their thought process rather than focusing solely on outcomes. This refined our way of measuring quality—CHP's consistency and adherence to optimum performance—gave them an opportunity to address key drivers. Furthermore, reliability measurement engaged the frontline in the identification of barriers and empowered them to actively participate in the development of solutions. Development and measurement of care bundles at CHP is an excellent high-yield process improvement example resulting from their benchmarking exercise.

Communication with SPS member hospitals encouraged CHP to review the connection between patient care policies and EHR-enabled care bundles. Before engagement with SPS, CHP was not reliably measuring adherence to their patient care policies. As discussed with the SPS network group, creation of a bundle began with identification of the 4 to 6 actions they need to consistently perform to prevent 95% of the HACs. These critical actions are then grouped into a measurable bundle or care plan. SPS philosophy served to educate member institutions to

1. Develop operational definition of HAC or event
2. Develop bundle (critical actions)
3. Develop the measurement of the bundle
4. Submit and share narratives: the process, barriers, and new knowledge

Participating hospitals quickly learned that the sharing component of SPS is an extraordinarily high-yield activity. Using the benchmarking process, CHP was able to identify areas in need of improvement regarding serious safety events. With comparative data at their disposal, CHP was able to target specific areas of interest,

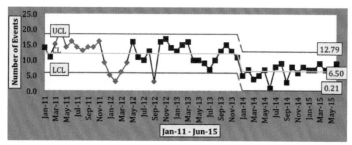

Fig. 2. Reduction in serious harm safety events 2011 to 2015. LCL, lower control limit; UCL, upper control limit.

appropriately trend and record the data, and compare findings with their peers to determine a best practice approach. An example of this effectiveness is the post-SPS engagement 55% reduction in serious safety events. Before engagement with SPS, CHP averaged approximately 14.4 serious safety events per month. Following engagement and process improvement with care bundles, they have reduced this to approximately 6.5 events per month and have been holding steady with this number since early 2014. A control chart of this improvement is noted in **Fig. 2**.

Directly complementary to their reduction in serious safety events, CHP recognized the need for improvement in organizational reporting culture.[16] For several years before SPS engagement, just culture has been a strategic priority for CHP; however, a focused communication campaign was needed to encourage staff to report near misses and other unsafe conditions. Staff members were educated on the importance of documenting and reporting events without fear of repercussion or punishment.

Overall, CHP has seen a consistent and steady increase in the reporting of events since their involvement in the collaborative, particularly in the area of medical education/residency trainees. Their dialogue with member hospitals, in conjunction with a sharpened focus on serious safety events, HACs, and adherence to bundles, has increased the reliability of the care they provide. Staff engagement with just culture has resulted in an increase in all-cause reported safety events, as noted in **Fig. 3**.

Engagement with SPS, in conjunction with continued focus on just culture within CHP yields an increase in available data. In turn, this translates into more accurate and reliable measurements due to the broader (greater numbers of areas reporting)

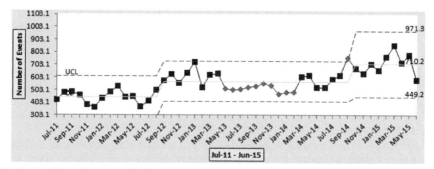

Fig. 3. Number of reported safety events (all cause). UCL, Upper Control Limit.

and larger overall sample size. This approach helped create an environment that furthers the culture of data-driven decision making within CHP.

SUMMARY

Consistent with the vision for safe, effective pediatric health care led by the AHRQ, engagement with the SPS collaborative has served to strengthen and reinforce CHP's core values of safe, highest-value pediatric care, consistently focused on the needs of their patients and families. In the words of a nursing leader at CHP, the SPS-engaged HAC teamwork "made measurement real." The knowledge of CHP's performance relative to their peer network serves as a catalyst for CHP to bolster their process improvement methodology. Recent successes in reduction of serious harm events, coupled with an increase in reported patient safety events, are evidence of this effectiveness.

Critical success factors before engagement include robust data sources, broad analytical training for leaders in statistical process control, and baseline work on just culture. Through this process, CHP's own culture of transparency has improved, with the knowledge that only by refining their internal reporting culture will they be able to make the changes necessary to improve their externally facing metrics. Current and future projects inspired by and complementary to the SPS HAC workgroups include the construction of pathways of care in the EHR as well as projects in patient/family discharge planning and education. Through benchmarking and collaboration with other member hospitals, CHP and SPS will continue to measure their journey toward the safest, highest-value care for children.

REFERENCES

1. Available at: www.qualityindicators.ahrq.gov. Accessed November, 2015.
2. NQI development. Available at: www.ahrq.gov. Accessed November, 2015.
3. Knapp JF, Hall M, Sharma V. Benchmarks for the emergency department care of children with asthma, bronchiolitis, and croup. Pediatr Emerg Care 2010;26(5): 364–9.
4. Available at: www.solutionsforpatientsafety.org/about-us. Accessed November, 2015.
5. Slonim AD, LaFleur BJ, Ahmed W, et al. Hospital-reported medical errors in children. Pediatrics 2003;111(3):617–21.
6. Pediatric quality indicators overview AHRQ quality indicators. Rockville (MD): Agency for Healthcare Research and Quality; 2006.
7. Centers for Medicare and Medicaid Services (CMS), HHS. Medicare program; hospital inpatient prospective payment systems for acute care hospitals and the long-term care hospital prospective payment system policy changes and fiscal year 2016 rates; revisions of quality reporting requirements for specific providers, including changes related to the electronic health record incentive program; Extensions of the Medicare-dependent, small rural hospital program and the low-volume payment adjustment for hospitals. Fed Regist 2015; 80(158):49325–886.
8. O'Brien A, Weaver C, Settergren TT, et al. EHR documentation: the hype and the hope for improving nursing satisfaction and quality outcomes. Nurs Adm Q 2015; 39(4):333–9.
9. Krasowski MD, Schriever A, Mathur G, et al. Use of a data warehouse at an academic medical center for clinical pathology quality improvement, education, and research. J Pathol Inform 2015;6:45.

10. Kirkendall ES, Goldenhar LM, Simon JL, et al. Transitioning from a computerized provider order entry and paper documentation system to an electronic health record: expectations and experiences of hospital staff. Int J Med Inform 2013; 82(11):1037–45.
11. Abraham J, Jerome-D'Emilia B, Begun JW. The diffusion of magnet hospital recognition. Health Care Manage Rev 2011;36(4):306–14.
12. Fretheim A, Tomic O. Statistical process control and interrupted time series: a golden opportunity for impact evaluation in quality improvement. BMJ Qual Saf 2015;24(12):748–52.
13. Mastro KA, Flynn L, Preuster C. Patient- and family-centered care: a call to action for new knowledge and innovation. J Nurs Adm 2014;44(9):446–51.
14. Brownlee K, Minnier TE, Martin SC, et al. A paradigm shift toward system wide quality improvement education: meeting the needs of a rapidly changing health care environment: meeting the needs of a rapidly changing health care environment. Qual Manag Health Care 2013;22(1):25–35.
15. Pattison J, Kline T. Facilitating a just and trusting culture. Int J Health Care Qual Assur 2015;28(1):11–26.
16. Ruddy RM, Chamberlain JM, Mahajan PV, et al, Pediatric Emergency Care Applied Research Network. Near misses and unsafe conditions reported in a Pediatric Emergency Research Network. BMJ Open 2015;5(9):e007541.

Electronic Health Record– Enabled Research in Children Using the Electronic Health Record for Clinical Discovery

Scott M. Sutherland, MD[a,b,]*, David C. Kaelber, MD, PhD, MPH[c],
N. Lance Downing, MD[b], Veena V. Goel, MD[a,b],
Christopher A. Longhurst, MD, MS[d]

KEYWORDS

- EHR • EMR • Electronic health record • Electronic medical record • Research
- Clinical discovery • Children

KEY POINTS

- The electronic health record (EHR) contains a massive amount of discrete patient data that are generated through the routine provision of patient care.
- EHR data can be so-called big data based on volume (total number of patients/data points), velocity (the rate at which it is generated), and/or variety.
- Data validation is imperative because many of the data were collected for clinical, rather than research, purposes.
- EHR data can be used to build large patient cohorts and/or identify patients with rare conditions, allowing pediatric researchers to overcome small samples sizes.
- The EHR can be used for interventional studies and prospective trials at the point of care.

Disclosure: None of the authors have anything to disclose.
[a] Department of Pediatrics, Stanford University School of Medicine, 300 Pasteur Drive, Room G-306, Stanford, CA 94304, USA; [b] Department of Clinical Informatics, Stanford Children's Health, 1265 Welch Road, MSOB XIC65A, Stanford, CA 94305, USA; [c] Departments of Information Services, Internal Medicine, Pediatrics, Epidemiology and Biostatistics, Center for Clinical Informatics Research and Education, The MetroHealth System, Case Western Reserve University, 2500 MetroHeatlh Drive, Cleveland, OH 44109, USA; [d] Department of Biomedical Informatics, UC San Diego School of Medicine, 9560 Towne Centre Drive, San Diego, CA 92121, USA
* Corresponding author. 300 Pasteur Drive, Room G-306, Stanford, CA 94304.
E-mail address: suthersm@stanford.edu

Pediatr Clin N Am 63 (2016) 251–268
http://dx.doi.org/10.1016/j.pcl.2015.12.002
0031-3955/16/$ – see front matter © 2016 Elsevier Inc. All rights reserved.

pediatric.theclinics.com

INTRODUCTION

Although electronic health records (EHRs) were first described more than 50 years ago, it is only recently that EHRs have become pervasive.[1] Notably, the Unites States saw EHR adoption triple between 2009 and 2013; adoption among children's hospitals increased from 21% in 2008 to 59% in 2011.[2,3] The growth seen over the last 5 years is likely to be progressive and sustainable as, with time, countries such as Norway, the Netherlands, New Zealand, and the United Kingdom have achieved near-universal EHR adoption.[4] As experience with EHRs has increased, clinicians and researchers have begun to see the EHR in a different light; as a colossal database and interventional tool at the intersection of physicians, patients, and care delivery.[5,6] In the past, research databases, tools, and records have been separate from clinical databases, tools, and records; EHRs blur these distinctions and merge these silos.

In parallel with increased EHR adoption, there has been the evolution of clinical informatics, the "scientific and medical field that concerns itself with the cognitive, information processing and communication tasks of medical practice, education and research, including the information science and the technology to support these tasks."[7] More specifically, clinical research informatics, which generates the tools and techniques to use the EHR for clinical research, has been developed within the larger field of clinical informatics.[8]

The combination of increased EHR implementation, the exponential growth of digital data available within the EHR, and the development of clinical research informatics tools and techniques present a unique, previously unavailable opportunity to enhance clinical discovery and improve patient care. This phenomenon has particular relevance in children's health care. Pediatric research often involves small samples sizes[9]; by exploiting the EHR data sets across 1 or more institutions, investigators have access to a vast number of patients and can mitigate concerns about statistical power and significance. In addition, when faced with clinical decisions, pediatricians are often forced to rely on studies and trials that have been performed in adults; trials are often not repeated in children because of cost, safety, and redundancy issues.[10] EHR data can be used to retrospectively assess the impact of clinical decisions, making it possible to determine the efficacy of a certain intervention or the safety of a particular medication. In addition, when pediatric trials are implemented, they are often hampered by slow recruitment and erratic referrals.[11] The EHR can be used to facilitate recruitment for trials across institutions and improve the efficacy of trial procedures.[4,12] It is within this context that this article presents an overview of EHR-enabled clinical discovery, focusing on concepts and studies relevant to pediatrics.

THE ELECTRONIC HEALTH RECORD DATA SET

The EHR data set is immense; the scale is on par with many of the big data disciplines such as genomics and proteomics. Across an entire children's hospital, clinical care generates hundreds of thousands of data points per day and tens of millions of data points annually; data generated from ambulatory care and the narrative data contained within clinical notes add substantially more information. However, although the volume of data is alluring, some elements are easier to extract, some have higher fidelity, and some require validation.[13] Thus, an understanding of the types and quality of data available is essential to using EHRs for clinical discovery.

Electronic Health Record Data Elements

The EHR contains clinical data generated through the routine provision of care: physician orders, test results, vital signs, demographics, progress notes, medication administration data, and so forth. Depending on the institution, it may include financial, operational, and technical information. Some data are discrete (vital signs), some are textual (progress notes), and some are scanned (medical records from outlying facilities). Although some elements conform to national ontology standards (eg, Common Procedural Terminology [CPT]; International Classification of Diseases 9, Clinical Modification [ICD-9-CM/ICD-10-CM]; Systematized Nomenclature for Medicine [SNO-MED], Unified Medical Language System [UMLS]), many are locally defined.[14] **Table 1** shows typical types of data present in most EHRs and an assessment of their quality.

Electronic Health Record Data Validation/Corroboration

Although validating data is always important, it is especially critical when analyzing large EHR data sets in which the data may have been collected for clinical rather than research purposes. There are 2 main methodological approaches to corroborate potential findings. One common approach is internal validation, which typically involves a detailed, manual evaluation of a random subset (sometimes only 1% or less) of the large data set to determine fidelity.[15] The other primary approach is external validation. Here findings are corroborated by other studies or data from a different data source; findings that are consistent with previous studies or alternate

| **Table 1** | | |
| **Qualitative assessment of EHR data quality** | | |
Type of Data	Relative Quality	Comments
Demographic (eg, age, gender)	Very high	EHRs overestimate the number/percentage of patients who are alive because of limited processes to update patients' statuses unless they expire in the hospital
Laboratory results (eg, LOINC codes)	Very high	Data collected for clinical and not research purposes so sometimes a laboratory test was never ordered that would have been ideal; a laboratory result that does not exist is not the same as a negative laboratory result
Prescriptions/ medications ordered (eg, RX-Norm codes)	Very high	In some cases, up to 31% of prescriptions written are not filled[67]
Vital signs	High	Data collected for clinical and not research purposes
Test orders	High	Most EHRs have provider order entry; orders can be used as a surrogate to understand provider thought process, intent, and sometime diagnoses even if the test is never completed or results are unavailable
Diagnoses (eg, ICD-9/ICD-10 codes)	Medium	Highly variable; probably higher sensitivity, but lower specificity for rarer, more serious diseases
Family history, social history, past medical and surgical history (eg, ICD-9/ICD-10; CPT codes)	Low	Often missing; high if data collection is mandated and standardized, such as smoking status for ages 13 y and older
Other	Unknown	Many other data elements exist in EHRs; need to understand qualitatively and quantitatively EHR variables that you want to use

Abbreviation: LOINC, logical observation identifiers names and codes.

data sources are more likely to be correct.[16] Of note, if the finding of interest is a relative difference between groups whose data come from the same source, validation may be less critical as long as obvious biases are not apparent between the groups.[17] In addition, because larger data sets make it statistically easier to find statistically significant results that may not be clinically significant (or even clinically plausible), a biological plausibility hypothesis should exist for findings and hypotheses should be developed before data analysis begins.

ELECTRONIC HEALTH RECORD–ENABLED RESEARCH METHODOLOGIES AND EXAMPLES OF ANALYTICAL APPROACHES

The types of studies that can be performed using EHR data typically conform to the fairly standard methodologies used with other types of data. A summary of these approaches and their advantages/disadvantages in clinical research informatics is shown in **Table 2**. Detailed in **Table 3** is a comprehensive list, by study type, of EHR-enabled pediatric studies as of publication.

Electronic Health Record–enabled Retrospective, Observational Research

Retrospective, observational studies that take advantage of the size of the EHR data set are perhaps the most common type of EHR-enabled research. Although hypotheses are generated and analytics are applied retrospectively, the data are collected prospectively in real-time as patient care is delivered; patients receive interventions/therapies and undergo monitoring in a nonexperimental fashion according to locally

Table 2
Special EHR research design methodologies

Research Methodology	Advantages	Disadvantages	Comments
Retrospective cohort/ case-control study	• Leverages increased historical EHR • Fewer resources to collect	• Clinical data not collected for research purposes so may be of more variable quality • Desired data may be missing	Population level, deidentified data do not need IRB approval
Before-after technology intervention	For large implementations (such as implementing e-prescribing in a practice or health care system) no other methodology may be possible	Could be unrecognized temporal confounders	—
Randomized cluster control trial	Reduces individual bias or cross-contamination from patient-based or provider-based randomization	Depending on EHR, may be technically difficult to implement	A cluster would be a group of providers or single site

Abbreviation: IRB, institutional review board.

Table 3
EHR-enabled pediatric studies

Title of Article	Investigators
Retrospective, Observational Studies	
Diabetes Mellitus Screening in Pediatric Primary Care	Anand et al,[68] 2006
The Natural History of Weight Percentile Changes in the First Year of Life	Bennett et al,[33] 2014
Trends in the Diagnosis of Overweight and Obesity in Children and Adolescents: 1999–2007	Benson et al,[26] 2009
Screening for Obesity-related Complications Among Obese Children and Adolescents: 1999–2008	Benson et al,[15] 2011
Development of Heart and Respiratory Rate Percentile Curves for Hospitalized Children	Bonafide et al,[28] 2013
Low-pressure Valves in Hydrocephalic Children: A Retrospective Analysis	Breimer et al,[69] 2012
Association Between Maintenance Fluid Tonicity and Hospital-acquired Hyponatremia	Carandang et al,[27] 2013
Heart Rates in Hospitalized Children by Age and Body Temperature	Daymont et al,[30] 2015
Evaluation of the Quality of Antenatal Care Using Electronic Health Record Information in Family Medicine Clinics of Mexico City	Doubova et al,[70] 2014
Identifying Factors Predicting Immunization Delay for Children Followed in an Urban Primary Care Network Using an Electronic Health Record	Fiks et al,[71] 2006
Impact of Immunization at Sick Visits on Well-child Care	Fiks et al,[72] 2008
Association of Late-preterm Birth with Asthma in Young Children: Practice-based Study	Goyal et al,[73] 2011
Underdiagnosis of Hypertension in Children and Adolescents	Hansen et al,[25] 2007
Increased Prevalence of Eosinophilic Gastrointestinal Disorders in Pediatric PTEN Hamartoma Tumor Syndromes (PHTS)	Henderson et al,[24] 2014
Real-time Forecasting of Pediatric Intensive Care Unit Length of Stay Using Computerized Provider Orders	Levin et al,[50] 2012
Comparison of New Modeling Methods for Postnatal Weight in ELBW Infants Using Prenatal and Postnatal Data	Porcelli & Rosenbloom,[31] 2014
Specialized Pediatric Growth Charts for Electronic Health Record Systems: The Example of Down Syndrome	Rosenbloom et al,[32] 2010
AKI in Hospitalized Children: Epidemiology and Clinical Associations in a National Cohort	Sutherland et al,[48] 2013
AKI in Hospitalized Children: Comparing the pRIFLE, AKIN, and KDIGO Definitions	Sutherland et al,[74] 2015
Retinopathy of Prematurity in English Neonatal Units: A National Population-based Analysis Using NHS Operational Data	Wong et al,[19] 2013

(continued on next page)

Table 3
(continued)

Title of Article	Investigators
Interventional Quality-improvement Studies and Trials	
Computerized Physician Order Entry with Decision Support Decreases Blood Transfusions in Children	Adams et al,[35] 2011
Automated Primary Care Screening in Pediatric Waiting Rooms	Anand et al,[44] 2012
Advanced Clinical Decision Support for Vaccine Adverse Event Detection and Reporting	Baker et al,[75] 2015
Improved Documentation and Care Planning with an Asthma-specific History and Physical	Beck et al,[76] 2012
Impact of a Computerized Template on Antibiotic Prescribing for Acute Respiratory Infections in Children and Adolescents	Bourgeois et al,[77] 2010
Improving Immunization Delivery Using an Electronic Health Record: The ImmProve Project	Bundy et al,[78] 2013
Use of a Computerized Decision Aid for ADHD Diagnosis: A Randomized Controlled Trial	Carroll et al,[46] 2013
Use of a Computerized Decision Aid for Developmental Surveillance and Screening: A Randomized Clinical Trial	Carroll et al,[45] 2014
Impact of Real-time Electronic Alerting of Acute Kidney Injury on Therapeutic Intervention and Progression of RIFLE Class	Colpaert et al,[40] 2012
Recognizing Hypoglycemia in Children Through Automated Adverse-event Detection	Dickerman et al,[79] 2011
Impact of Clinical Alerts Within an Electronic Health Record on Routine Childhood Immunization in an Urban Pediatric Population	Fiks et al,[80] 2007
Impact of Electronic Health Record-based Alerts on Influenza Vaccination for Children with Asthma	Fiks et al,[37] 2009
Improving Adherence to Otitis Media Guidelines with Clinical Decision Support and Physician Feedback	Forrest et al,[81] 2013
Electronic Health Record Identification of Nephrotoxin Exposure and Associated Acute Kidney Injury	Goldstein et al,[39] 2013
Developing Clinical Decision Support Within a Commercial Electronic Health Record System to Improve Antimicrobial Prescribing in the Neonatal ICU	Hum et al,[82] 2014
Development and Performance of Electronic Acute Kidney Injury Triggers to Identify Pediatric Patients at Risk for Nephrotoxic Medication-associated Harm	Kirkendall et al,[83] 2014
A Quality Improvement Project to Improve Compliance with the Joint Commission Children's Asthma Care-3 Measure	Kuhlmann et al,[84] 2013
Development of a Web-based Decision Support Tool to Increase Use of Neonatal Hyperbilirubinemia Guidelines	Longhurst et al,[41] 2009
Using Electronic Health Record Alerts to Provide Public Health Situational Awareness to Clinicians	Lurio et al,[85] 2010

Impact of a Clinical Decision Support System on Antibiotic Prescribing for Acute Respiratory Infections in Primary Care: A Quasi-Experimental Trial	Mainous et al, [86] 2013
Optimizing Care of Adults with Congenital Heart Disease in a Pediatric Cardiovascular ICU Using Electronic Clinical Decision Support	May et al, [38] 2014
Embedding Time-limited Laboratory Orders Within Computerized Provider Order Entry Reduces Laboratory Utilization	Pageler et al, [43] 2013
Use of Electronic Medical Record-enhanced Checklist and Electronic Dashboard to Decrease CLABSIs	Pageler et al, [42] 2014
Impact of Electronic Medical Record Integration of a Handoff Tool on Sign-out in a Newborn Intensive Care Unit	Palma et al, [87] 2011
Integrating the Home Management Plan of Care for Children with Asthma into an Electronic Medical Record	Patel et al, [88] 2012
Integrating of Clinical Decision Support with On-line Encounter Documentation for Well Child Care at the Point of Care	Porcelli & Lobach, [89] 1999
Childhood Obesity: Can Electronic Medical Records Customized with Clinical Practice Guidelines Improve Screening and Diagnosis?	Savinon et al, [90] 2012
Putting Guidelines into Practice: Improving Documentation of Pediatric Asthma Management Using a Decision-making Tool	Shapiro et al, [91] 2011
Optimization of Drug-Drug Interaction Alert Rules in a Pediatric Hospital's Electronic Health Record System Using a Visual Analytics Dashboard	Simpao et al, [92] 2015
Developing and Evaluating a Machine Learning Based Algorithm to Predict the Need of Pediatric Intensive Care Unit Transfer for Newly Hospitalized Children	Zhai et al, [47] 2014
Improving Home Management Plan of Care Compliance Rates Through an Electronic Asthma Action Plan	Zipkin et al, [93] 2013
Prospective Trials and Studies	
Electronic Health Record-based Decision Support to Improve Asthma Care: A Cluster-randomized Trial	Bell et al, [36] 2010
A Shared E-decision Support Portal for Pediatric Asthma	Fiks et al, [94] 2014
Adoption of Electronic Medical Record-based Decision Support for Otitis Media in Children	Fiks et al, [95] 2015
Comparative Effectiveness of Childhood Obesity Interventions in Pediatric Primary Care: A Cluster-randomized Clinical Trial	Taveras et al, [65] 2015

derived standards of care.[18] A few pediatric practices and health care systems have had robust EHRs in place for more than 15 years, creating important opportunities to perform retrospective, cohort, and case-control studies using existing EHR data. Given the current trend toward increased EHR adoption, the impact of these studies is likely to expand significantly over time; a recent study from the United Kingdom, where EHR adoption is nearly universal, was able to pool data from 94% of all the neonatal units across the country.[19]

One way to leverage EHR data is to extract and manipulate them to create immense data sets. These data sets may be big based on their volume (eg, total number of patients), their velocity (the rate at which data are generated; eg, vital signs monitors now generate many data points per patient per day), and/or their variety (types of data available, including sources previously unavailable, such as environmental data or patient-entered data). Once a hypothesis has been determined and a research strategy identified, the process required to create these data sets can be laborious (**Fig. 1**). Data are stored within the EHR in a manner that optimizes data entry and patient-level data display. However, this is not always conducive to clinical discovery and

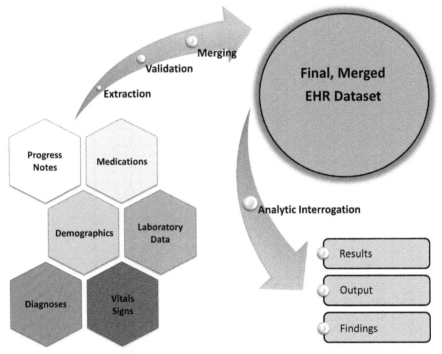

Fig. 1. EHR-enabled data extraction, validation, and analysis. Use of EHR data for research purposes requires several interconnected processes. Data are extracted from the EHR; careful attention must be paid to determine which elements are required in order to optimize analytical success and minimize personal health information–related risk. Once extracted, the data must be cleaned and validated. Validated data elements are merged into a unified database through various linking identifiers. This database can then be subjected to analytical interrogation. Various groups have begun to centralize this process (electronic Pediatric Research in Office Settings [ePROS] and Comparative Effectiveness Research through Collaborative Electronic Reporting [CER²]), integrating data from multiple EHRs into a consolidated data warehouse.

analytics.[20] Different data elements for the same patient are often stored in different areas of the EHR; the elements must be extracted individually and then merged using a linking identifier such as a medical record number. In addition, the data must be interrogated, standardized, normalized, and validated before analysis. Although these challenges are surmountable, it is important to understand the process when interpreting EHR data and research. Development of similarly sized data sets prospectively in a more controlled fashion would be time and resource prohibitive; although the EHR data require extraction and manipulation, their generation and acquisition are fully funded through the delivery of clinical care. Several groups have taken a consolidative, centralized approach to address this issue, integrating retrospective data from multiple EHRs. Probably the most robust example of this is the Comparative Effectiveness Research through Collaborative Electronic Reporting (CER^2) Consortium, which was recently established by the American Academy of Pediatrics (AAP) Pediatric Research in Office Settings (PROS).[21,22] The AAP's electronic PROS (ePROS) EHR data network, which was established in 2010, is now also integrated with the CER^2 collaborative to improve the health of children and enhance primary care practice by conducting and fostering national collaborative practice-based research using EHR systems.[23] CER^2 has been tasked with developing a multisite EHR collaborative that will serve as the platform for EHR-enabled pharmacoepidemiologic studies, as successfully demonstrated by the proof-of-concept retrospective studies on psychotropic and asthma medication[24] use and side effects. By providing access to EHR clinical data for more than 1.4 million pediatric primary care patients, this collaborative group will benefit from economies of scale in making EHR data more accessible to researchers.

One example of EHR-enabled retrospective, observational research examined ambulatory hypertension across a cohort of nearly 15,000 children.[25] Although 507 (3.6%) children met criteria for hypertension, only 131 of those (26%) were ever diagnosed with hypertension; nearly three-quarters of pediatric hypertension was missed. A similar study examined obesity diagnosis trends across more than 60,000 children and found that overweight, obesity, and severe obesity were also underdiagnosed.[26] A third example evaluated the association between administration of hypotonic maintenance fluid and the subsequent development of hyponatremia in hospitalized children.[27] This study created the largest such cohort to date and was able to confirm that hypotonic fluids are associated with an increased risk of hyponatremia.

EHR data can also be used to generate or optimize normative data. At present, many of the available pediatric normative data are derived from generalized cohorts of healthy, ambulatory children; data on hospitalized children are sparse.[28,29] In 2013, Bonafide and colleagues[28] used nurse-documented vital signs across more than 14,000 pediatric hospitalizations at 2 major children's hospitals to generate heart rate and respiratory rate percentiles for hospitalized children. Their values were significantly different than the normative data currently in use, which could have a serious impact on optimized vital sign parameters, alerts, and assessment of pediatric inpatients. Daymont and colleagues[30] in 2015 used EHR-documented vital sign data to the relationship between EHR and body temperature. Similar studies have harnessed the EHR data set to derive growth curves for extremely low birthweight infants and children with trisomy 21, as well as to describe the natural history of weight percentile changes in the first year of life.[31–33]

Data from within EHRs can also be used to identify and study rare conditions. Although a provider may have seen 1 or 2 cases of an uncommon disease, the number of patients seen across the institution might be 10-fold higher, and the number of patients seen across a multi-institution collaborative might be 100-fold higher.

EHR-enabled research is able to rely on the collective, enduring memory of the institution, which has the potential to dramatically increase case yield. This approach was used to study plastic bronchitis in children; an uncommon and poorly reported disease.[34] By sifting through more than 200,000 pediatric patients at a single institution, 14 children were identified, which made it possible to describe the epidemiology, pathologic findings, and successful treatment strategies. Similarly, interrogation of a cohort of more than 1 million children enabled researchers to confirm a hypothetical association between eosinophilic gastrointestinal disorders and the PTEN hamartoma tumor syndromes (PHTS), two rare and previously unassociated conditions.[24]

A special case of EHR-enabled, retrospective observational studies is the use of deidentified, population-level EHR data. Aggregated, normalized sets of EHR data containing millions of pediatric patients now exist, along with the tools necessary to query such data. These data sets and tools can be used for certain types of research and may be more efficient and provide more statistical power than traditional research studies. One such example studied risk factors for venous thrombosis using a retrospective EHR data set spanning 13 years and nearly 1 million patients.[16] The findings corroborated those of a prospective study that was conducted over 14 years; for comparative purposes, the EHR-enabled study, which examined almost 50 times as many patients, was completed over 11 weeks and required input from only 5 individuals. A similar technique was used to investigate the untoward side effects associated with azathioprine administration; across nearly 15,000 patients receiving azathioprine (culled from a population of >10 million), neutropenia was common but hepatotoxicity was unassociated with azathioprine use.[17] It is possible that this methodology could become a new standard for postmarket drug surveillance; this would have important ramifications for pediatricians because such studies are not performed prospectively in children with the same regularity as in adults.

Electronic Health Record–enabled Quality Improvement and Assessment of Interventional Impact

In addition to functioning as the data repository for clinical care delivery, the EHR offers a platform for intervention. Practitioners can integrate clinical decision support into the EHR in a myriad of ways: best practice advisories, quality improvement bundles, diagnostic tools, research findings, and even predictive algorithms. As an example, Adams and colleagues[35] combined decision support and computerized physician order entry to reduce inappropriate transfusion frequency. By alerting clinicians to relevant, consensus guidelines at the point of order entry, the intervention resulted in a statistically significant reduction in red blood cell usage without a negative impact on other patient safety outcomes. Other similar examples of interventional informatics include the use of decision support tools to improve care of children with asthma and adults with congenital heart disease[36–38]; to prevent acute kidney injury progression, neonatal hyperbilirubinemia, central line infections, and laboratory test overuse[39–43]; and to target outpatient screening for developmental surveillance, vaccination eligibility, and attention-deficit/hyperactivity disorder.[44–46]

The EHR also has the potential to predict and prevent adverse outcomes and severe disease. The temporal nature of EHR data allows clinicians to anchor an event in time, creating a clear delineation between pre-event data and postevent data. The pre-event data can then be used to derive a predictive algorithm. These prediction models can based on institutional experience, known disease-related risk factors, or even high-content, high-throughput machine learning techniques.[47,48] This approach can be used to predict prolonged intensive care unit length of stay, pediatric emergency department crowding, sepsis, cardiovascular decompensation, and even death in real time.[49,50]

Electronic Health Record–enabled Prospective Research

Increasing prospective trial costs have fueled interest in identifying ways to make clinical research more efficient, which has encouraged the use of clinical registries to perform comparative effectiveness research.[6,51,52] However, although retrospective data analysis is effective, prospective, randomized controlled trials (RCTs) are the gold standard for experimental research.[53] Recent evidence has shown that the EHR represents a powerful tool capable of making prospective research more affordable.[12,54] Although regulatory and ethical issues remain critical topics, these EHR-enabled RCTs represent a disruptive technology that is able to reduce trial costs by leveraging existing infrastructure and clinical data collection.[55]

Although several applications of EHR-enabled prospective research have been described, one of the most practical has been the ability to enhance trial recruitment.[6,56] Given the myriad of discrete data elements contained within the EHR, automated identification of potential trial recipients requires only the integration of inclusion and exclusion filters; the EHR can then single out patients as they meet the predetermined criteria.[57,58] In pediatrics, 2 distinct approaches have been used.[59] The first approach uses a pop-up alert for clinicians; physicians are notified at the point of care that the patient is eligible for enrollment. The second approach involves the automated creation of a patient list; these EHR-derived lists are provided to trial recruiters who can approach potential participants separately.[59] In the arena of pediatric trials, in which study power and sample sizes are at a premium, any improvement in patient identification is likely to improve enrollment.

Although identification of eligible cohorts is an attractive use of clinical registries and EHRs, some informaticists have taken this one step further by using the EHR to conduct RCTs at the point of care. The Thrombus Aspiration in ST-Elevation Myocardial Infarction trial used the existing work flow and data collection mechanisms of the national Swedish Angiography and Angioplasty Registry platform to randomize 5000 patients with myocardial infarctions.[60] Coordinators consented patients after the diagnosis had been confirmed and used an automated randomization module within the registry to assign patients to either thrombus aspiration plus percutaneous coronary intervention (PCI) or PCI alone. Researchers were able to achieve a 100% follow-up rate, streamline data capture, all at an incremental cost of $50 per patient. The Study of Access Site for Enhancement of Percutaneous Coronary Intervention for Women similarly used existing registry infrastructure to reduce data acquisition costs in a randomized trial comparing femoral versus radial access for PCI; registry integration led to a 65% reduction in coordinator workload.[61] Moving beyond an EHR-enabled registry, the direct use of the EHR can improve efficiency and efficacy even further. One such point-of-care clinical trial (POCCT) comparing 2 insulin regimens used the Veteran Administration's EHR; an alert giving the option to enroll in the trial was delivered to clinicians in real time when they entered an order for insulin.[62] Important operational considerations for EHR POCCTs include research-specific billing, the use of a patient portal for patient-reported outcomes, integration of case report forms into the EHR, and the reliability of existing EHR data. Each of these topics merits careful consideration and further study. Although these trials highlight the potential of EHR-enabled prospective research, issues of clinical equipoise, ethics, work flow burden, and informed consent must be addressed.[63,64] Of note, to date there are no studies in the literature of which the authors are aware that use the EHR as the intervention and the tool to facilitate an RCT in pediatrics.[65]

LIMITATIONS SURROUNDING ELECTRONIC HEALTH RECORD–ENABLED RESEARCH

EHR-enabled research and the data contained within the EHR offer several benefits. However, this methodology is subject to certain limitations. Most fundamentally, other than studies that use the EHR to facilitate prospective trials, using EHR data to enable clinical discovery is retrospective and observational in nature. Although many interesting associations can be identified, retrospective studies cannot prove causality. Some clinicians think of EHR-enabled inquiry as hypothesis generating rather than hypothesis proving; EHR-enabled studies should not replace RCTs. One particularly difficult aspect is the potential for bias and confounding. As clinical care is delivered, patient factors and provider preferences affect both treatment decisions and outcomes; retrospectively, it can be challenging to eliminate such biases. In addition, it can be difficult to determine and control for disease severity retrospectively; researchers need to be diligent and creative in their efforts to address bias and confounding.

Other limitations include missing or flawed data. In certain situations, EHR work flow does not effectively capture data elements; for example, heights are rarely recorded on patients admitted to the intensive care unit. Certain techniques can be used to impute missing data; however, these methods are not as reliable as possessing the data themselves. Flawed data can be more problematic to address. It can be difficult to determine when a weight has been mistakenly entered in pounds instead of kilograms or a decimal point has been moved 1 digit to the left. However, given the size of the data sets generated by this technique, unless the data are systematically flawed, most such errors tend to have marginal impact on the results because of the overall regression to the mean effect. Additional issues with data fidelity include the analysis of unstructured data that are currently limited by text analytics algorithms such as natural language processing.[66]

In addition, although clearly a strength, there are times when the scale of the data available can be problematic. As seen in **Fig. 1**, different elements are stored in different data tables; the different tables may have different formats or even different identifier elements. Thus, EHR data are not stored in a manner that is necessarily conducive to research. Extracting and linking the data can be time and labor intensive. Manipulation and analysis of the data can, at times, require high-content, high-throughput techniques. However, with the appropriate personnel in place, this is a limitation that can be overcome.

SUMMARY

EHRs are becoming integrated into the fabric of children's health and are critical to the future of clinical discovery. EHR-enabled research offers great potential; as EHR adoption expands, the possibilities of EHR-enabled clinical discovery will increase substantially. The capacity to generate vast retrospective cohorts and big data–sized data sets is one of the most practical applications of the technique. However, as clinicians come to better understand the intersection between the EHR, care delivery, clinical and translational research, and quality improvement, the use of the EHR as a platform for care improvement and outcomes research is likely to become more innovative. With time, it is possible that EHR-enabled research will allow clinicians to enhance scientific investigation, learn from every patient at every visit, deliver high-quality clinical decision support in real time at the point of care, and reach the goal of achieving a true learning health care environment.

REFERENCES

1. Schenthal JE, Sweeney JW, Nettleton W Jr. Clinical application of electronic data processing apparatus. II. New methodology in clinical record storage. JAMA 1961;178(3):267–70.
2. Nakamura MM, Harper MB, Jha AK. Change in adoption of electronic health records by US children's hospitals. Pediatrics 2013;131(5):e1563–75.
3. Charles D, King J, Patel V, et al. Adoption of electronic health record systems among U.S. non-federal acute care hospitals: 2008-2012. Washington, DC: Office of the National Coordinator for Health Information Technology; 2013. ONC Data Brief, no 9.
4. Schoen C, Osborn R, Squires D, et al. A survey of primary care doctors in ten countries shows progress in use of health information technology, less in other areas. Health Aff 2012;31(12):2805–16.
5. Frankovich J, Longhurst CA, Sutherland SM. Evidence-based medicine in the EMR era. N Engl J Med 2011;365(19):1758–9.
6. Longhurst CA, Harrington RA, Shah NH. A 'Green Button' for using aggregate patient data at the point of care. Health Aff 2014;33(7):1229–35.
7. Greenes RA, Shortliffe EH. Medical informatics: an emerging academic discipline and institutional priority. JAMA 1990;263(8):1114–20.
8. Embi PJ, Payne PRO. Clinical research informatics: challenges, opportunities and definition for an emerging domain. J Am Med Inform Assoc 2009;16(3):316–27.
9. van der Tweel I, Askie L, Vandermeer B, et al. Standard 4: determining adequate sample sizes. Pediatrics 2012;129(Suppl 3):S138–45.
10. Bourgeois FT, Murthy S, Pinto C, et al. Pediatric versus adult drug trials for conditions with high pediatric disease burden. Pediatrics 2012;130(2):285–92.
11. Caldwell PH, Butow PN, Craig JC. Parents' attitudes to children's participation in randomized controlled trials. J Pediatr 2003;142(5):554–9.
12. Antman EM, Harrington RA. Transforming clinical trials in cardiovascular disease: mission critical for health and economic well-being. JAMA 2012;308(17):1743–4.
13. Wasserman RC. Electronic medical records (EMRs), epidemiology, and epistemology: reflections on EMRs and future pediatric clinical research. Acad Pediatr 2011;11(4):280–7.
14. Spooner SA, Classen DC. Data standards and improvement of quality and safety in child health care. Pediatrics 2009;123(Suppl 2):S74–9.
15. Benson LJ, Baer HJ, Kaelber DC. Screening for obesity-related complications among obese children and adolescents: 1999–2008. Obesity 2011;19(5):1077–82.
16. Kaelber DC, Foster W, Gilder J, et al. Patient characteristics associated with venous thromboembolic events: a cohort study using pooled electronic health record data. J Am Med Inform Assoc 2012;19(6):965–72.
17. Patel VN, Kaelber DC. Using aggregated, de-identified electronic health record data for multivariate pharmacosurveillance: a case study of azathioprine. J Biomed Inform 2014;52:36–42.
18. Gallego B, Dunn AG, Coiera E. Role of electronic health records in comparative effectiveness research. J Comp Eff Res 2013;2(6):529–32.

19. Wong HS, Santhakumaran S, Statnikov Y, et al. Retinopathy of prematurity in English neonatal units: a national population-based analysis using NHS operational data. Arch Dis Child Fetal Neonatal Ed 2013;99(3):F196–202.

20. Schneeweiss S. Learning from big health care data. N Engl J Med 2014;370(23): 2161–3.

21. American Academy of Pediatrics Department of Research. Research ADo. AAP research network to use data in electronic health records. AAP News 2012; 33(7):16.

22. Fiks AG, Grundmeier RW, Steffes J, et al. Comparative effectiveness research through a collaborative electronic reporting consortium. Pediatrics 2015;136(1): e215–24.

23. Boss RD. Ethics for the pediatrician: pediatric research ethics: evolving principles and practices. Pediatr Rev 2010;31(4):163–5.

24. Henderson CJ, Ngeow J, Collins MH, et al. Increased prevalence of eosinophilic gastrointestinal disorders in pediatric PTEN hamartoma tumor syndromes. J Pediatr Gastroenterol Nutr 2014;58(5):553–60.

25. Hansen ML, Gunn PW, Kaelber DC. Underdiagnosis of hypertension in children and adolescents. JAMA 2007;298(8):874–9.

26. Benson L, Baer HJ, Kaelber DC. Trends in the diagnosis of overweight and obesity in children and adolescents: 1999-2007. Pediatrics 2009;123(1):e153–8.

27. Carandang F, Anglemyer A, Longhurst CA, et al. Association between maintenance fluid tonicity and hospital-acquired hyponatremia. J Pediatr 2013;163(6): 1646–51.

28. Bonafide CP, Brady PW, Keren R, et al. Development of heart and respiratory rate percentile curves for hospitalized children. Pediatrics 2013;131(4):e1150–7.

29. Fleming S, Thompson M, Stevens R, et al. Normal ranges of heart rate and respiratory rate in children from birth to 18 years of age: a systematic review of observational studies. Lancet 2011;377(9770):1011–8.

30. Daymont C, Bonafide CP, Brady PW. Heart rates in hospitalized children by age and body temperature. Pediatrics 2015;135(5):e1173–81.

31. Porcelli PJ, Rosenbloom YT. Comparison of new modeling methods for postnatal weight in ELBW infants using prenatal and postnatal data. J Pediatr Gastroenterol Nutr 2014;59(1):E2–8.

32. Rosenbloom ST, McGregor TL, Chen Q, et al. Specialized pediatric growth charts for electronic health record systems: the example of Down syndrome. AMIA Annu Symp Proc 2010;2010:687–91.

33. Bennett WE Jr, Hendrix KS, Thompson RT, et al. The natural history of weight percentile changes in the first year of life. JAMA Pediatr 2014;168(7):681–2.

34. Kunder R, Kunder C, Sun HY, et al. Pediatric plastic bronchitis: case report and retrospective comparative analysis of epidemiology and pathology. Case Rep Pulmonol 2013;2013:8.

35. Adams ES, Longhurst CA, Pageler N, et al. Computerized physician order entry with decision support decreases blood transfusions in children. Pediatrics 2011; 127(5):e1112–9.

36. Bell LM, Grundmeier R, Localio R, et al. Electronic health record–based decision support to improve asthma care: a cluster-randomized trial. Pediatrics 2010; 125(4):e770–7.

37. Fiks AG, Hunter KF, Localio AR, et al. Impact of electronic health record-based alerts on influenza vaccination for children with asthma. Pediatrics 2009;124(1): 159–69.

38. May LJ, Longhurst CA, Pageler NM, et al. Optimizing care of adults with congenital heart disease in a pediatric cardiovascular ICU using electronic clinical decision support. Pediatr Crit Care Med 2014;15(5):428–34.
39. Goldstein SL, Kirkendall E, Nguyen H, et al. Electronic health record identification of nephrotoxin exposure and associated acute kidney injury. Pediatrics 2013; 132(3):e756–67.
40. Colpaert K, Hoste EA, Steurbaut K, et al. Impact of real-time electronic alerting of acute kidney injury on therapeutic intervention and progression of RIFLE class. Crit Care Med 2012;40(4):1164–70.
41. Longhurst C, Turner S, Burgos AE. Development of a web-based decision support tool to increase use of neonatal hyperbilirubinemia guidelines. Jt Comm J Qual Patient Saf 2009;35(5):256–62.
42. Pageler NM, Longhurst CA, Wood M, et al. Use of electronic medical record–enhanced checklist and electronic dashboard to decrease CLABSIs. Pediatrics 2014;133(3):e738–46.
43. Pageler NM, Franzon D, Longhurst CA, et al. Embedding time-limited laboratory orders within computerized provider order entry reduces laboratory utilization. Pediatr Crit Care Med 2013;14(4):413–9.
44. Anand V, Carroll AE, Downs SM. Automated primary care screening in pediatric waiting rooms. Pediatrics 2012;129(5):e1275–81.
45. Carroll AE, Bauer NS, Dugan TM, et al. Use of a computerized decision aid for developmental surveillance and screening: a randomized clinical trial. JAMA Pediatr 2014;168(9):815–21.
46. Carroll AE, Bauer NS, Dugan TM, et al. Use of a computerized decision aid for ADHD diagnosis: a randomized controlled trial. Pediatrics 2013;132(3):e623–9.
47. Zhai H, Brady P, Li Q, et al. Developing and evaluating a machine learning based algorithm to predict the need of pediatric intensive care unit transfer for newly hospitalized children. Resuscitation 2014;85(8):1065–71.
48. Sutherland SM, Ji J, Sheikhi FH, et al. AKI in hospitalized children: epidemiology and clinical associations in a national cohort. Clin J Am Soc Nephrol 2013;8(10): 1661–9.
49. Bouleux G, Marcon E, Mory O. Early index for detection of pediatric emergency department crowding. IEEE J Biomed Health Inform 2015;19(6):1929–36.
50. Levin SR, Harley ET, Fackler JC, et al. Real-time forecasting of pediatric intensive care unit length of stay using computerized provider orders. Crit Care Med 2012; 40(11):3058–64.
51. Fiks AG, Grundmeier RW, Margolis B, et al. Comparative effectiveness research using the electronic medical record: an emerging area of investigation in pediatric primary care. J Pediatr 2012;160(5):719–24.
52. Luce BR, Kramer JM, Goodman SN, et al. Rethinking randomized clinical trials for comparative effectiveness research: the need for transformational change. Ann Intern Med 2009;151(3):206–9.
53. Benson K, Hartz AJ. A comparison of observational studies and randomized, controlled trials. N Engl J Med 2000;342(25):1878–86.
54. Vickers AJ, Scardino PT. The clinically-integrated randomized trial: proposed novel method for conducting large trials at low cost. Trials 2009;10:14.
55. Lauer MS, D'Agostino RB. The randomized registry trial — the next disruptive technology in clinical research? N Engl J Med 2013;369(17):1579–81.
56. Simpson LA, Peterson L, Lannon CM, et al. Special challenges in comparative effectiveness research on children's and adolescents' health. Health Aff 2010; 29(10):1849–56.

57. Hawkins MS, Hough LJ, Berger MA, et al. Recruitment of veterans from primary care into a physical activity randomized controlled trial: the experience of the VA-STRIDE study. Trials 2014;15:11.

58. Navaneethan SD, Jolly SE, Sharp J, et al. Electronic health records: a new tool to combat chronic kidney disease? Clin Nephrol 2013;79(3):175–83.

59. Grundmeier RW, Swietlik M, Bell LM. Research subject enrollment by primary care pediatricians using an electronic health record. AMIA Annu Symp Proc 2007;2007:289–93.

60. Fröbert O, Lagerqvist B, Olivecrona GK, et al. Thrombus aspiration during ST-segment elevation myocardial infarction. N Engl J Med 2013;369(17):1587–97.

61. Hess CN, Rao SV, Kong DF, et al. Embedding a randomized clinical trial into an ongoing registry infrastructure: unique opportunities for efficiency in design of the Study of Access site For Enhancement of Percutaneous Coronary Intervention for Women (SAFE-PCI for Women). Am Heart J 2013;166(3):421–8.e421.

62. D'Avolio L, Ferguson R, Goryachev S, et al. Implementation of the Department of Veterans Affairs' first point-of-care clinical trial. J Am Med Inform Assoc 2012; 19(e1):e170–6.

63. Faden RR, Beauchamp TL, Kass NE. Informed consent, comparative effectiveness, and learning health care. N Engl J Med 2014;370(8):766–8.

64. Magnus D, Caplan AL. Risk, consent, and support. N Engl J Med 2013;368(20): 1864–5.

65. Taveras EM, Marshall R, Kleinman KP, et al. Comparative effectiveness of childhood obesity interventions in pediatric primary care: a cluster-randomized clinical trial. JAMA Pediatr 2015;169(6):535–42.

66. Barrett N, Weber-Jahnke JH. Applying natural language processing toolkits to electronic health records - an experience report. Stud Health Technol Inform 2009;143:441–6.

67. Tamblyn R, Eguale T, Huang A, et al. The incidence and determinants of primary nonadherence with prescribed medication in primary care: a cohort study. Ann Intern Med 2014;160(7):441–50.

68. Anand SG, Mehta SD, Adams WG. Diabetes mellitus screening in pediatric primary care. Pediatrics 2006;118(5):1888–95.

69. Breimer GE, Sival DA, Hoving EW. Low-pressure valves in hydrocephalic children: a retrospective analysis. Childs Nerv Syst 2012;28(3):469–73.

70. Doubova SV, Perez-Cuevas R, Ortiz-Panozo E, et al. Evaluation of the quality of antenatal care using electronic health record information in family medicine clinics of Mexico City. BMC Pregnancy Childbirth 2014;14:168.

71. Fiks AG, Alessandrini EA, Luberti AA, et al. Identifying factors predicting immunization delay for children followed in an urban primary care network using an electronic health record. Pediatrics 2006;118(6):e1680–6.

72. Fiks AG, Hunter KF, Localio AR, et al. Impact of immunization at sick visits on well-child care. Pediatrics 2008;121(5):898–905.

73. Goyal NK, Fiks AG, Lorch SA. Association of late-preterm birth with asthma in young children: practice-based study. Pediatrics 2011;128(4):e830–8.

74. Sutherland SM, Byrnes JJ, Kothari M, et al. AKI in hospitalized children: comparing the pRIFLE, AKIN, and KDIGO definitions. Clin J Am Soc Nephrol 2015;10(4):554–61.

75. Baker MA, Kaelber DC, Bar-Shain DS, et al. Advanced clinical decision support for vaccine adverse event detection and reporting. Clin Infect Dis 2015;61(6): 864–70.

76. Beck AF, Sauers HS, Kahn RS, et al. Improved documentation and care planning with an asthma-specific history and physical. Hosp Pediatr 2012;2(4):194–201.
77. Bourgeois FC, Linder J, Johnson SA, et al. Impact of a computerized template on antibiotic prescribing for acute respiratory infections in children and adolescents. Clin Pediatr 2010;49(10):976–83.
78. Bundy DG, Persing NM, Solomon BS, et al. Improving immunization delivery using an electronic health record: the ImmProve project. Acad Pediatr 2013;13(5):458–65.
79. Dickerman MJ, Jacobs BR, Vinodrao H, et al. Recognizing hypoglycemia in children through automated adverse-event detection. Pediatrics 2011;127(4):e1035–41.
80. Fiks AG, Grundmeier RW, Biggs LM, et al. Impact of clinical alerts within an electronic health record on routine childhood immunization in an urban pediatric population. Pediatrics 2007;120(4):707–14.
81. Forrest CB, Fiks AG, Bailey LC, et al. Improving adherence to otitis media guidelines with clinical decision support and physician feedback. Pediatrics 2013;131(4):e1071–81.
82. Hum RS, Cato K, Sheehan B, et al. Developing clinical decision support within a commercial electronic health record system to improve antimicrobial prescribing in the neonatal ICU. Appl Clin Inform 2014;5(2):368–87.
83. Kirkendall ES, Spires WL, Mottes TA, et al. Development and performance of electronic acute kidney injury triggers to identify pediatric patients at risk for nephrotoxic medication-associated harm. Appl Clin Inform 2014;5(2):313–33.
84. Kuhlmann S, Mason B, Ahlers-Schmidt CR. A quality improvement project to improve compliance with the joint commission children's asthma care-3 measure. Hosp Pediatr 2013;3(1):45–51.
85. Lurio J, Morrison FP, Pichardo M, et al. Using electronic health record alerts to provide public health situational awareness to clinicians. J Am Med Inform Assoc 2010;17(2):217–9.
86. Mainous AG, Lambourne CA, Nietert PJ. Impact of a clinical decision support system on antibiotic prescribing for acute respiratory infections in primary care: quasi-experimental trial. J Am Med Inform Assoc 2013;20(2):317–24.
87. Palma JP, Sharek PJ, Longhurst CA. Impact of electronic medical record integration of a handoff tool on sign-out in a newborn intensive care unit. J Perinatol 2011;31(5):311–7.
88. Patel SJ, Longhurst CA, Lin A, et al. Integrating the home management plan of care for children with asthma into an electronic medical record. Jt Comm J Qual Patient Saf 2012;38(8):359–65.
89. Porcelli PJ, Lobach DF. Integration of clinical decision support with on-line encounter documentation for well child care at the point of care. Proc AMIA Symp 1999;599–603.
90. Saviñon C, Taylor JS, Canty-Mitchell J, et al. Childhood obesity: can electronic medical records customized with clinical practice guidelines improve screening and diagnosis? J Am Acad Nurse Pract 2012;24(8):463–71.
91. Shapiro A, Gracy D, Quinones W, et al. Putting guidelines into practice: Improving documentation of pediatric asthma management using a decision-making tool. Arch Pediatr Adolesc Med 2011;165(5):412–8.
92. Simpao AF, Ahumada LM, Desai BR, et al. Optimization of drug-drug interaction alert rules in a pediatric hospital's electronic health record system using a visual analytics dashboard. J Am Med Inform Assoc 2015;22(2):361–9.

93. Zipkin R, Schrager SM, Keefer M, et al. Improving home management plan of care compliance rates through an electronic asthma action plan. J Asthma 2013;50(6):664–71.

94. Fiks AG, Mayne S, Karavite DJ, et al. A shared e-decision support portal for pediatric asthma. J Ambul Care Manage 2014;37(2):120–6.

95. Fiks AG, Zhang P, Localio AR, et al. Adoption of electronic medical record-based decision support for otitis media in children. Health Serv Res 2015;50(2): 489–513.

Quality Care and Patient Safety in the Pediatric Emergency Department

Johanna R. Rosen, MD[a],*, Srinivasan Suresh, MD, MBA[b], Richard A. Saladino, MD[a]

KEYWORDS

- Pediatric emergency care • Quality improvement
- Quality improvement frameworks and methodology • Performance measures

KEY POINTS

- During the 15 years since the Institute of Medicine report on errors in medical care, quality improvement and patient safety have become priorities in health care.
- Process and quality improvement should guide safe, effective, efficient, timely, patient-centered, and equitable care to patients.
- The framework of the Institute of Medicine's domains of healthcare quality, the Donabedian categories, and the Acute Care Model all provide blueprints for change.

THE INSTITUTE OF MEDICINE'S CALL FOR IMPROVEMENT

During the last 15 years, quality improvement (QI) moved to the forefront of medical care in the United States. This focus started with the Institute of Medicine (IOM) report *To Err is Human: Building a Safer Health System*.[1] The IOM report described the many lives affected, and dollars lost, by flaws in health care systems.

A subsequent publication from the IOM defined quality as the degree to which health services for individuals and populations increase the likelihood of desired health outcomes and are consistent with current professional knowledge.[2] The IOM described 6 aims of quality to pursue in all health care settings:

- Effective: provide services based on scientific knowledge to all who can benefit and refrain from providing services to those not likely to benefit (avoiding underuse and overuse)

Disclosures: None.
[a] Division of Pediatric Emergency Medicine, Department of Pediatrics, Children's Hospital of Pittsburgh, University of Pittsburgh School of Medicine, 4401 Penn Avenue, AOB 2nd Floor, Suite 2400, Pittsburgh, PA 15224, USA; [b] Children's Hospital of Pittsburgh, 4401 Penn Avenue, Room 6415 AOB, Pittsburgh, PA 15224, USA
* Corresponding author.
E-mail address: Johanna.Rosen@chp.edu

Pediatr Clin N Am 63 (2016) 269–282
http://dx.doi.org/10.1016/j.pcl.2015.12.004
0031-3955/16/$ – see front matter © 2016 Elsevier Inc. All rights reserved.

- Safe: avoid injuries to patients from the care that is intended to help them
- Efficient: avoid waste, in particular waste of equipment, supplies, ideas, and energy
- Timely: reduce sometimes harmful delays for both those who receive and those who give care
- Equitable: provide care that does not vary in quality because of personal characteristics such as gender, ethnicity, geographic location, and socioeconomic status
- Patient-centered: provide care that is respectful of, and responsive to, individual patient preferences, needs, and values and ensure that patient values guide all clinical decisions

In response to the call by the IOM for improvement in health care, the American College of Graduate Medical Education and the American Board of Pediatrics now require training and participation in QI work. It is important to recognize that, in the short term, many of those charged with teaching quality and safety science do not have formal training. Therefore, rapid acquisition of such science is required of all who answer the call of the IOM.

QUALITY IMPROVEMENT FRAMEWORKS

At present, taking on the challenge of improving health care quality in a pediatric emergency department (ED) presents unique hurdles inherent to emergency care. Mahajan,[3] from Children's Hospital of Michigan, summarized the complexity of the chaotic ED setting, including the occurrence of multiple distractions (competing patient care priorities), incomplete information (some children present without family members to provide histories), and increasing ED patient volumes in many institutions in the United States. The IOM recognizes and draws attention to EDs being at a breaking point in these regards.

In an attempt to help bridge the gap between pediatric emergency medicine providers' general lack of formal training in QI methodology and the expectation that pediatric emergency medicine providers be responsible for improving the quality of care in pediatric EDs, Dr Mahajan[3] reviewed QI frameworks, terms, and tools inherent to QI methodology.

Three frameworks enable clinicians to understand, address, and evaluate QI efforts:

1. The IOM's 6 domains of health care quality
2. Donabedian's[4] quality framework
3. The Acute Care Model

The 6 domains of health care quality, as developed and described by the IOM, and listed earlier are effective, safe, efficient, timely, equitable, and patient-centered care. Categorizing QI endeavors into these domains is widely accepted and understood in the QI medical community. Many QI efforts cross categories. For example, improving the process to reduce pain in children with acute fractures addresses effective care, timely care, and patient-centered care.

The Donabedian[4] quality framework categorizes QI work into 3 groups:

1. Structure: the setting of care, including physical layout of the ED and available resources
2. Process: the patient experience in the ED, such as pathway-guided care
3. Outcomes: includes morbidity and mortality but also includes many other measures, such as frequency of antibiotic use or time metrics

The Donabedian categories are interrelated. Resources in play and the processes experienced by the patient may determine the outcome for a specific episode of care. The example of improving process to reduce pain in children with acute fractures is within the Process Donabedian framework, but affects the Outcome category as well.

The Acute Care Model was developed by Iyer and colleagues[5] to address the complexity of a pediatric ED and to focus QI efforts. The model facilitates a detailed understanding of existing systems and helps to uncover areas of improvement, especially for ED flow. The Acute Care Model calls for adoption of a common language and an effort to improve 4 integrated components of acute care:

1. Segmentation: patient triage based on severity of illness or injury. Several triage scores are used widely. For example, a common system is the 5-level tool called the Emergency Severity Index (ESI).[6] The ESI is a validated ED triage score based on predicted resource consumption and length of stay in the department. In addition, several trauma scores are used to anticipate staffing and resources needed for patients with traumatic injuries.
2. Therapeutic reliability: safe and effective treatment is provided in a timely manner and in a way that prevents deterioration. For example, an ED may have processes in place that prioritize a rapid response and provision of evidence-based therapies that optimize outcome for patients with asthma, anaphylaxis, or hyperbilirubinemia.
3. Diagnostic accuracy: a correct diagnosis is made in a safe, effective, and efficient manner, particularly when a patient presents with undifferentiated illness.
4. Disposition: correct disposition to home, hospital, or intensive care unit (ICU), or transfer to other facility is made with accuracy, minimizing return visits.

The Acute Care Model tracks each patient through the ED visit, from initial segmentation to disposition, with consideration of diagnostic accuracy and therapeutic reliability as often as needed. The model helps to frame and organize QI work in pediatric emergency medicine beyond the level of process mapping (examples of Acute Care Model organization are given in Ref.[5]). In brief, the model can be used to create pathways for clinically apparent illnesses with high illness severity, low variability in treatment, and high probability of admission, such as neonates with fever, children with severe asthma exacerbations, and febrile children with short gut syndrome or cancer.

Iyer and colleagues[5] also describe core competencies required for the Acute Care Model to be successfully applied in emergency medicine QI:

1. Appropriate segmentation of patients
2. Appropriate and rigorous use of evidence for diagnostic accuracy and for therapeutic reliability
3. Care systems with an emphasis on high reliability: preoccupation with failure, sensitivity to operations, resiliency, reluctance to simplify, and deference to expertise
4. Organizational leadership that supports and sustains a culture of improvement by:
   a. Clearly communicating goals
   b. Sharing data transparently
   c. Providing system support that helps ED staff accomplish the stated goals
   d. Imposing clear consequences when goals are not achieved

QUALITY IMPROVEMENT METHODS AND TOOLS

Methods used for QI vary based on the setting and desired outcomes. For pediatric emergency medicine, the Model for Improvement reference is the book by Langley and colleagues.[6,7] This model asks 3 fundamental questions, followed by tests of change with plan-do-study-act (PDSA) cycles.

1. What needs to be accomplished? That is, what is the purpose, goal, or aim of the project?
2. How can it be determined that a change is an improvement? That is, what will be measured to show improvement (or lack of improvement)? There are 3 categories of measurement to be considered:
   a. Outcome measures: for example, reduction in pain score after early provision of a pain medication
   b. Process measures: for example, time from patient arrival to the provision of a pain medication
   c. Balance measures: an unexpected outcome, such as prolonged ED length of stay
3. What change can be made that will result in an improvement? That is, what is the change idea to be tested?

The Model for Improvement can incorporate lessons learned from the process improvement approaches taken by high reliability organizations such as Six-sigma and Lean.

Briefly, Six-sigma process improvement methods organize the development of process improvement strategies into the DMAIC (define, measure, analyze, improve, and control) methodology to reduce variation[3]:

- Define the problem
- Measure by collecting data
- Analyze the data and brainstorm solutions
- Improve the process by applying ideas
- Control performance by monitoring improvement

Lean process improvement methods focus on:

- Improved workflow
- Reducing waste
- Maximizing value-added processes

Again, once these sorts of methods are used, tests of change are then made by incorporating the PDSA cycle (discussed later).

SPECIFIC TOOLS FOR QUALITY IMPROVEMENT

Tools used in QI pursuits include process maps, failure modes and effects analyses (FMEAs), Pareto charts, key driver diagrams, PDSA cycles, run charts, and control charts. These tools help to identify specific areas for improvement, keep the plan focused, and track changes over time.

Process mapping is a process by which a problem is identified and a multidisciplinary group convenes to map the process around that problem. This can also be done by direct observation of the process, not only from the perspective of the patient, but also from the perspectives of involved health care providers. Typically, mapping of an entire process reveals elements of the process that may be enhanced or eliminated to improve overall performance.

An **FMEA** provides annotation to a process map by identifying elements of process that are at risk of failure (what could go wrong), identifying potential causes of a failure (why this could go wrong), and the consequences of the failure (what may happen if this goes wrong). Members of a multidisciplinary team ask themselves these 3 questions for each step in the process, and then identify possible interventions to reduce the occurrence of the failure. This tool helps the team plan a process improvement project by choosing 1 or a few possible interventions on which to act, and recording the outcomes as the project moves forward.[7]

Pareto charts help QI teams prioritize possible interventions that may improve a process. Using baseline data, frequencies of failure are charted in order to provide a visual representation of the elements of the process to prioritize for change. Mahajan[3] identified elements of a patient hand-off process that were often missing or not well communicated and found that although patient identifiers and history were most often included in the hand-offs, the information about consultants and special clinical equipment needs were not as frequently included. Using a Pareto chart to show the higher frequency of these two elements of failure, focused education could then be used to improve the patient hand-off process.

Key driver diagrams are another commonly used tool to help focus quality and process improvement efforts (**Fig. 1**). A key driver diagram states the aim of the project and then lists all of the key drivers of the process. Key drivers are the factors that need to be in place in order for the aim to be achieved. Possible interventions are then identified to ensure that the key drivers are used in the process.

The QI tool for testing change ideas is the **PDSA cycle**. A QI work group may initiate a small-scale change with a limited group of patients or involving a few providers, and then conduct a PDSA cycle. The following is a description of each phase of the cycle[8]:

Plan:
- What is the question being asked? What change idea is being tested?
- What does the team predict will happen?
- Determine who, what, when, and where for the test and for the data collection.

Do:
- Perform the change, and collect data.
- In addition to planned data collection, keep track of observations not predicted or expected.

Study:
- Analyze the data, compare with predictions.

Act:
- Three next steps are options that are based on the results of the test:
  1. Adapt: improve the change and move on to a next PDSA cycle.
  2. Adopt: select the change for implementation on a larger scale.
  3. Abandon: discard this change idea.

To follow progress over time, QI teams use run charts and control charts. Run charts simply display the rate of an outcome, process, or balance measure over time (**Fig. 2**). They are annotated with PDSA cycles or other changes that may have occurred over time. They are used to help clinicians understand whether a particular intervention (or PDSA cycle) made a difference in the process measures and are often used to communicate progress to stakeholders.

Control charts are run charts that include control limits, or acceptable ranges in variation. With the addition of control limits, teams can determine whether variation in the results is common cause variation (acceptable variation in the process) or special cause variation (variation that is unlikely to occur by chance alone).

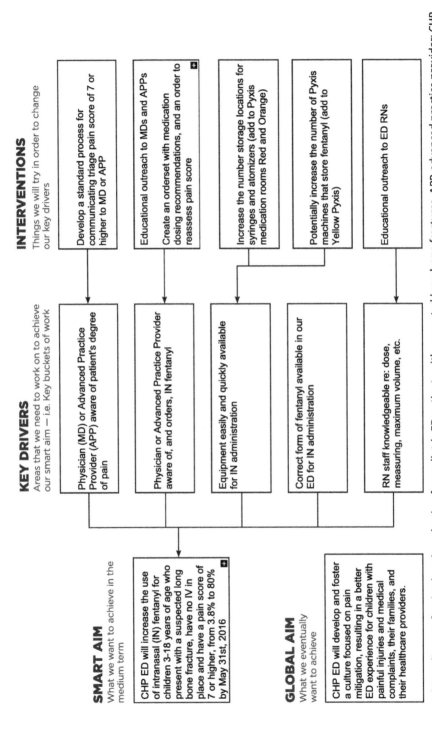

Fig. 1. Key driver diagram for timely pain reduction for pediatric ED patients with suspected long bone fractures. APP, advanced practice provider; CHP, Children's Hospital of Pittsburgh; ED, emergency department; IN, intranasal; IV, intravenous; MD, Doctor of Medicine; RN, registered nurse.

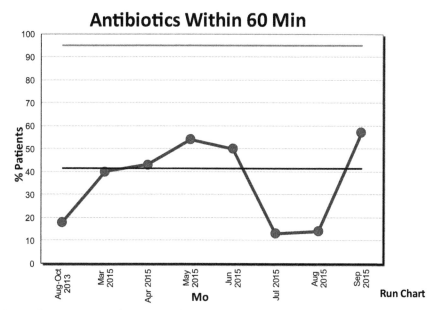

Fig. 2. The percentage of patients with presumed septic shock who receive their first dose of antibiotic within 60 minutes of recognition. The line at 41% is the median, and the line at 95% is the goal. This graph presents incomplete data from CHP ED, for illustration purposes only.

EVIDENCE-BASED GUIDELINES AND THEIR ROLE IN QUALITY CARE

Process mapping, organizing systems into the Acute Care Model, and review of control charts bring to light the variability of care in nearly every health care environment. Variability in health care results in variability of patient outcomes. In an effort to reduce variation in medical care, many pediatric EDs have a library of clinical pathways or evidence-based guidelines (EBGs). Some systems include automatic alerts, often called best practice alerts (BPAs), to remind physicians to consider a certain diagnosis and related evaluation based on patient data that are available in the electronic medical record. The ultimate goal of EBGs and BPAs is to translate evidence into bedside practice.[9]

In response to the concerns that EBGs reflect so-called cookbook medicine that ignores patient individuality or are too complex to easily integrate into daily practice, Chumpitazi and colleagues[9] state that carefully developed EBGs should help health care providers reduce the complexity of care, streamline processes, and allow allocation of time and resources to other and more complex patients. In addition, well-thought-out EBGs apply to approximately 80% of targeted patients, whereas 20% of patients require evaluation or treatment not outlined in an EBG (the Pareto 80/20 principle).

Chumpitazi and colleagues[9] describe focusing on 4 care processes while developing EBGs:

- Disease processes with a high prevalence
- Care processes with high variability in care delivery
- Diseases requiring high resource use
- Disease processes with high morbidity or mortality

EBG development requires interdisciplinary input and a thorough review of the literature to determine current best practices based on the best evidence. If evidence is lacking or equivocal, practitioners are encouraged to come to an agreement with advice from experts and to be transparent in the recommendations so that users of the guidelines understand the underpinnings of the advice.

The investigators also recognize and note that implementation of EBGs is difficult. Knowing how best to incorporate guidelines into everyday practice requires thought and input from all those who provide patient care. Process mapping is an especially important tool that can help in this regard.

MEASURING QUALITY IN PEDIATRIC EMERGENCY MEDICINE

Alessandrini and Knapp[10] describe quality metrics and performance measures that should be followed by all pediatric EDs to ensure quality care as defined by the IOM.[10] The ultimate purpose of measuring care and performance is to improve the care and enable good outcomes to be sustained. Measuring allows systems to inform patients, the public, and health care societies such as the American Academy of Pediatrics. Transparency of performance data builds trust within communities. Measuring also allows for incentive plans to be a part of motivating health care providers to provide the best evidence-based care.

Quality measures can be categorized into the IOM's 6 domains of health care quality and into the Donabedian Structure-Process-Outcome framework:

Timely care:
- Time from triage to physician evaluation (Donabedian Process)
- Time from triage to administration of intravenous fluids for children with diabetic ketoacidosis (Donabedian Process)
- Rate of children who left without being seen (Donabedian Outcome)

Effective care:
- Percentage of patients with postsedation discharge instructions (Donabedian Process)
- Forty-eight-hour readmission rate (Donabedian Outcome)

Efficient care:
- Percentage of patients with minor head trauma receiving a head computed tomography scan (Donabedian Process)
- Total ED length of stay (Donabedian Outcome)

Safe care:
- Proportion of patients without a documented weight (Donabedian Process)
- Proportion of patients without presedation airway assessment (Donabedian Process)
- Patients admitted to an inpatient unit, then transferred to an ICU within 12 hours (Donabedian Outcome)
- Adverse drug events (Donabedian Outcome)

Patient-centered care:
- Availability of translation services (Donabedian Structure)
- Reducing pain in children with acute fractures (Donabedian Outcome)
- Rate of patient complaints (Donabedian Outcome)

Equitable care:
- Income, ethnic, and geographic differences in immunization rate (Donabedian Outcome)

Alessandrini published work from a Targeted Issues Grant from the Emergency Medical Services for Children program called Defining Quality Performance Measures for Pediatric Emergency Care[11] as a response to the IOM's report, *Emergency Care for Children: Growing Pains*, which calls for the creation of national standards for pediatric emergency care.[12] The program details 60 performance measures related to pediatric emergency care. Fifteen of the 60 measures were determined to be top rated for testing and improvement based on:

1. Importance to emergency medical services for children
2. Scientific acceptability
3. Usability
4. Feasibility by a diverse stakeholder group that included pediatric emergency medical physicians, general emergency medical physicians practicing in academic or community settings, nurses, and parents

Examples of the top 15 quality measures for pediatric emergency medicine are:

1. Measuring weight in kilograms for patients less than 18 years of age
   a. IOM quality domains: Effective, Safe
   b. Donabedian framework: Process
2. Having pediatric equipment in the ED
   a. IOM quality domains: Effective, Safe
   b. Donabedian framework: Process
3. Time from door to provider
   a. IOM quality domains: Timely, Patient Centered
   b. Donabedian framework: Outcome
4. Reducing pain in children with acute fractures
   a. IOM quality domains: Effective, Timely, Patient Centered
   b. Donabedian framework: Process
5. Children with mild head trauma receiving a head computed tomography scan
   a. IOM quality domains: Safe, Efficient
   b. Donabedian framework: Process
6. Evidence-based guideline for bronchiolitis
   a. IOM quality domains: Effective, Efficient
   b. Donabedian framework: Structure
7. Reducing antibiotic use in children with viral illness
   a. IOM quality domains: Effective, Efficient
   b. Donabedian framework: Process
8. Return visits within 48 hours resulting in admission
   a. IOM quality domains: Effective, Efficient
   b. Donabedian framework: Process

LOCAL EXAMPLES OF QUALITY IMPROVEMENT WORK IN A PEDIATRIC EMERGENCY DEPARTMENT

At Children's Hospital of Pittsburgh, several quality-of-care improvements have been trialed in the ED. Three examples are provided.

Emergency Department Time-out Vital Signs Check

In 2004, after recognizing that children admitted from the ED sometimes acutely worsen on a hospital inpatient unit and have a significant clinical decline or an arrest event, we instituted a QI improvement process for review of time-out vital signs before transfer from the ED. After a child was determined to be ready for admission to the inpatient unit from the ED, a nurse measured and recorded a final set of vital signs and reviewed them with the ED attending of record. This final review was to serve as a safety net for patients for whom there may have been a recent untoward change in their vital signs. Should the final vital signs require an intervention, the patient was held in the ED until the vital signs were acceptable for transfer to the inpatient unit.

The data collected in a 2-year period following the institution of the QI intervention suggested a trend toward fewer arrest and clinical decline alerts called on inpatient units.[13] Just as importantly, anecdotally, many patients were held in the ED for additional treatment (eg, additional fluid bolus or respiratory treatment) as a result of the recognition of a change in clinical status or incomplete response to ED therapy. This intervention fits within the IOM domain of patient safety.

Emergency Department Screening for Sexually Transmitted Infection

In 2011, in partnership with the Children's Hospital of Pittsburgh Division of Adolescent Medicine, the authors recognized that there was an opportunity to improve the frequency of testing for sexually transmitted infections for adolescent girls with abdominal or urinary complaints.[14] At the time we were primarily using urine samples for *Chlamydia trachomatis* (CT) and gonorrhea (GC) testing; this was not state-of-the-art.

Vaginal self-swabs for CT and GC are more sensitive and specific for the detection of *Chlamydia* and gonorrhea than urine samples, and are the preferred method of testing for most adolescent girls.[15,16] The authors performed a root-cause analysis and found that our laboratory had the appropriate swabs, but that we did not regularly stock the swabs in our ED. An education intervention was initiated for ED nurses and attending physicians, as well as advanced practice providers, residents, and fellows. GC and CT swabs were routinely stocked in supply carts in each ED examination room, and we created an electronic order set to help standardize ordering of the testing. After these interventions, we increased the use of vaginal swabs from 6.6% (17 out of 256) to 69% (69 out of 100). This QI project is an example of effective medical care.

Emergency Department Management of Sexual Assault Referrals

Children's Hospital of Pittsburgh is a tertiary care referral center for children in western Pennsylvania, eastern Ohio, and northern West Virginia. Referrals for possible sexual assault occur each day, but not all of these children need to be seen in the ED.

The authors retrospectively tested and prospectively implemented a sexual assault triage tool developed by Floyd and colleagues[17] at Emory University. A closed-loop process was developed between our ED and our hospital Child Advocacy Center (CAC) specialists allowing for communication between the referring ED, the Children's Hospital ED staff, the patient and family, and our CAC staff. During a 1-year period after implementation of the screening tool, we received 36 referral calls. More than half of these patients (19 out of 36; 53%) were directed to nonemergent care. On review by the CAC staff, all of these 19 patients were appropriately screened and avoided unnecessary travel, expenses, and stress associated with an ED-to-ED transfer.[18] This improvement project is an example of effective, efficient, and patient-centered care, as described by the IOM.

COLLABORATIVE DEVELOPMENT OF SAFETY FOR CHILDREN AT RISK FOR SEPTIC SHOCK

A collaborative of hospitals working on QI initiatives in an effort to do QI may facilitate uptake of QI methodology, consensus building, and rapid dissemination of knowledge.

Our ED joined the American Academy of Pediatrics Pediatric Septic Shock Collaborative (PSSC) in 2013. This initiative was developed by the American Academy of

Pediatric Septic Shock Collaborative Trigger Tool

Septic Shock Criteria (see reverse for vital signs)

1. Fever or Hypothermia
2. Tachycardia
3. Tachypnea
4. *Hypotension*
5. Capillary refill abnormality: ≥3, <1 sec
6. Pulse abnormality: decreased, bounding
7. Skin abnormality: mottled, flushed, petechiae/purpura
8. Mental status abnorm: depressed, highly irritable, confused

Inclusion Criteria:

Hypotension -OR-

≥ **3 of 8** above clinical criteria -OR-

High-risk condition plus ≥ **2 of 8** above clinical criteria

High Risk Patients:

Age < 1m, Severe MR/CP, Immunocompromised, Transplant
Asplenia (including SCD), Central line, Malignancy

Vital Signs Rules:

Age	Temp (°C)	HR	RR	Systolic BP
0 d - 1 m	< 36.5 or > 38	> 205	> 60	< 60
≥ 1 m - 3 m	< 36 or > 38	> 205	> 60	< 70
≥ 3 m - 1 y	< 36 or > 38.5	> 190	> 60	< 70
1 y	< 36 or > 38.5	> 190	> 40	< 72
2 y	< 36 or > 38.5	> 140	> 40	< 74
3 y	< 36 or > 38.5	> 140	> 40	< 76
4 y	< 36 or > 38.5	> 140	> 34	< 78
5 y	< 36 or > 38.5	> 140	> 34	< 80
6 y	< 36 or > 38.5	> 140	> 30	< 82
7 y	< 36 or > 38.5	> 140	> 30	< 84
8 y	< 36 or > 38.5	> 140	> 30	< 86
9 y	< 36 or > 38.5	> 140	> 30	< 88
≥ 10 y - 13 y	< 36 or > 38.5	> 100	> 30	< 90
> 13 y	< 36 or > 38.5	> 100	> 20	< 90

If Patient Meets Septic Shock Criteria:

- Inform MD/RN of concern
- Implement Septic Shock Powerplan
- Move patient to the critical care area

Fig. 3. PSSC Trigger Tool with the 9 criteria for consideration when evaluating a patient for possible septic shock. The table shows age-specific vital sign thresholds. BP, blood pressure; CP, cerebral palsy; HR, heart rate (beats per minute); MR, mental retardation; RR, respiration rate (breaths per minute); SCD, sickle cell disease.

Pediatrics Section on Emergency Medicine Committee on Quality Transformation in 2011. EDs from 25 hospitals across the country work together to reduce morbidity and mortality from presumed septic shock. The aims include reducing mortality from septic shock by a relative 20% and to increase the number of patients who receive the first intravenous fluid bolus within 20 minutes of arrival by 20%.

Key drivers for this project include early recognition of septic shock and early escalation of care. Change strategies to address these key drivers include implementation of a triage trigger tool and a process by which a senior physician is involved in the care of each patient early in the ED visit. The triage trigger tool is composed of the 4 standard vital signs, 4 physical examination findings, and the presence of a high-risk condition, such as a central venous line or malignancy (**Fig. 3**). The criteria for presumed septic shock are based on recommendations from Pediatric Advanced Life Support and the Surviving Sepsis campaign. Each hospital incorporates the triage trigger tool in a way that fits into its standard practice. Most have chosen to incorporate it electronically as a best-practice alert.

Development of an electronic triage trigger tool and related alerts required collaboration with information technology. When the screening criteria are met, which detect a child at risk for septic shock, a lightning-bolt icon appears on the patient tracking board (**Fig. 4**). The icon is a visual cue for the attending physician assigned to that patient to evaluate the patient as soon as possible, and to determine whether or not to proceed with further evaluation for septic shock and aggressive management. To orient the clinicians with criteria of the triage trigger tool, we produced a badge tag that included the screening criteria and a chart of age-specific vital signs thresholds (see **Fig. 3**). These tags were distributed to all ED clinicians. In tandem, we developed a septic shock EBG to streamline care, and a standardized order set (a so-called power plan) to standardize and facilitate rapid treatment.

As part of the septic shock safety screening process, we follow several outcome, process, and balance measures:

- Outcome measures:
  - Mortality
  - Rapid transfers from floor to ICU (within 12 hours of admission)
  - ED visit 24 hours before visit of interest
- Process measures:
  - Compliance with initial clinical assessment (ie, full set of vitals within 30 minutes of arrival at the ED)

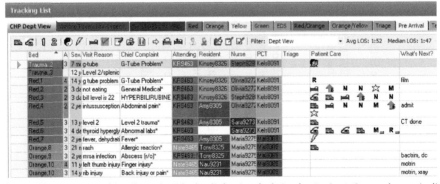

Fig. 4. ED patient tracking board with the lightning bolt in the Patient Care column, indicating the need for timely evaluation for possible septic shock (patient in bed 7).

- ○ First bolus within 20 minutes of recognition of septic shock risk
- ○ Antibiotics within 60 minutes of recognition of septic shock risk
- Balance measure:
  - ○ False-positives: patients who have a positive triage trigger tool, but are determined not to be appropriate for septic shock evaluation and treatment (eg, patient with asthma who presents with fever, tachycardia, and tachypnea)

Data are collected and submitted to the PSSC for full review and analysis across all the hospitals. The PSSC initiative is ongoing and data are shared during frequently scheduled collaborative-wide virtual meetings.

SUMMARY

During the 15 years since the IOM report, QI and patient safety have become priorities in health care. Process improvement and QI should guide safe, effective, efficient, timely, patient-centered, and equitable care to patients. The framework of the Institute of Medicine's quality care domains, the Donabedian categories, and the Acute Care Model all provide blueprints for change. Tools for change include the Model for Improvement, process maps, key driver diagrams, FMEAs, PDSA cycles, and EBGs. Experts in pediatric emergency medicine have at their disposal 60 quality performance measures, 15 of which are rated as top priorities.

ACKNOWLEDGMENTS

The authors thank the Pediatric Septic Shock Collaborative, American Academy of Pediatrics Section of Emergency Medicine, Committee on Quality Transformation, Caroline Vranesevic for design of the PSSC Trigger Tool Badge Tag.

REFERENCES

1. Institute of Medicine, Committee on Quality of Healthcare in America. To error is human: building a safer health system. Washington, DC: National Academies Press; 2000. Available at: http://www.nap.edu/catalog/9728/to-err-is-human-building-a-safer-health-system.
2. Institute of Medicine, Committee on Quality of Healthcare in America. Crossing the quality chasm: a new health system for the 21st century. Washington, DC: National Academies Press; 2001. Available at: http://www.nap.edu/catalog/10027/crossing-the-quality-chasm-a-new-health-system-for-the.
3. Mahajan P. Quality in pediatric emergency medicine: a learning curve and a curveball. Clin Pediatr Emerg Med 2011;12(2):80–90.
4. Donabedian A. Evaluating the quality of medical care. Milbank Mem Fund Q 1966;44(Suppl 3):166–206.
5. Iyer S, Reeves S, Varadarajan K, et al. The acute care model: a new framework for quality care in emergency medicine. Clin Pediatr Emerg Med 2011;12(2):91–101.
6. Emergency Severity Index. ESI Triage Algorithm. Available at: http://www.esitriage.org/. Accessed January 6, 2016.
7. Failure modes and effects analysis tool. Institute for Healthcare Improvement. 2014. Available at: http://www.ihi.org/resources/Pages/Tools/FailureModesandEffects AnalysisTool.aspx. Accessed November 20, 2015.
8. Langley GL, Moen R, Nolan KM, et al. The improvement guide: a practical approach to enhancing organizational performance. 2nd edition. San Francisco (CA): Jossey-Bass Publishers; 2009.

9. Chumpitazi CE, Barrera P, Macias CG. Diagnostic accuracy and therapeutic reliability in pediatric emergency medicine: the role of evidence based guidelines. Clin Pediatr Emerg Med 2011;12(2):113–20.

10. Alessandrini EA, Knapp J. Measuring quality in pediatric emergency care. Clin Pediatr Emerg Med 2011;12(2):102–12.

11. Top 15-rated hospital-based pediatric emergency care performance measures. Emergency Medical Services for Children National Resource Center. Available at: http://www.emscnrc.org/EMSC_Resources/ED_Pediatric_Performance_Measures_Toolbox.aspx. Accessed November 20, 2015.

12. Institute of Medicine, Committee on the Future of Emergency Care in the United States Health System, Board on Health Care Services. Emergency care for children: growing pains. Washington, DC: National Academies Press; 2007. Available at: http://www.nap.edu/catalog/11655/emergency-care-for-children-growing-pains.

13. Shah AP, Feidor-Hamilton M, Saladino RA, et al. Occurrence of inpatient condition A or C events after admission from a pediatric emergency department: effect of an "ED Time-Out Vital Sign Review" process. Platform presentation, American Academy of Pediatrics Annual Meeting. Abstract (#9980). San Francisco, October 1–5, 2010.

14. Kursmark M, Radovic A, Sieminski S, et al. Quality improvement intervention to improve testing for sexually transmitted infections in a pediatric emergency department. Abstract #755995, Publication #3365.5. Platform Presentation, Pediatric Academic Societies' 2013 Annual Meeting. May 4–7, 2013.

15. Schachter J, Chernesky MA, Willis DE, et al. Vaginal swabs are the specimens of choice when screening for *Chlamydia trachomatis* and *Neisseria gonorrhoeae*: results from a multicenter evaluation of the APTIMA assays for both infections. Sex Transm Dis 2005;32(12):725–8.

16. Chernesky MA, Hook EW 3rd, Martin DH, et al. Women find it easy and prefer to collect their own vaginal swabs to diagnose *Chlamydia trachomatis* or *Neisseria gonorrhoeae* infections. Sex Transm Dis 2005;32(12):729–33.

17. Floyed RL, Hirsch DA, Greenbaum VJ, et al. Development of a screening tool for pediatric sexual assault may reduce emergency department visits. Pediatrics 2011;128(2):221–6.

18. Horner KB, Fletcher K, Rosen JR, et al. Evaluation of a screening tool for sexual abuse referrals to the pediatric emergency department. Abstract #6. Poster presentation for American Academy of Pediatrics' National Conference and Exhibition. 2014. Available at: https://aap.confex.com/aap/2014/webprogrampress/Paper25268.html. Accessed November 20, 2015.

Patient Safety and Quality Metrics in Pediatric Hospital Medicine

Bhanumathy Kumar, MD

KEYWORDS

- Patient safety • Quality • Pediatric hospital medicine • Medical errors
- Multidisciplinary approach

KEY POINTS

- Patient safety is the responsibility of every health care provider.
- Because children cannot speak up for their own safety, pediatric health care workers have the added responsibility of being their advocates in promoting quality care that is, safe, effective, timely, readily accessible, and family friendly.
- Medical errors for the most part are related to system failures, such as equipment malfunction, communication breakdown, fragmented care, complex processes, and lack of standardized service.
- A multidisciplinary approach, communication, and teamwork are essential in providing high-quality care to patients, both during their hospitalization and after discharge.

INTRODUCTION

The implementation of quality control within the field of health care has become a matter of extreme importance in a very short period of time. From its initial surge of recognition less than 2 decades ago, standards of quality assurance have proliferated ceaselessly. These have been accompanied closely by intense scrutiny, and for good reason. Estimates of annual deaths due to medical errors have been placed in the hundreds of thousands. Errors in pediatric medicine are especially perturbing. Children are at a much higher risk of experiencing harm when compared with adults, mainly due to weight-based medication requirements, developmental changes, and dependency on caregivers.[1] Yet, pediatric quality measures still lag behind those of adults.

The author has nothing to disclose.
Department of Pediatrics, Children's Hospital of Michigan, Wayne State University, 3901 Beaubien Street, Detroit, MI 48201, USA
E-mail address: bkumar@dmc.org

Pediatr Clin N Am 63 (2016) 283–291
http://dx.doi.org/10.1016/j.pcl.2015.11.002
0031-3955/16/$ – see front matter Published by Elsevier Inc.

pediatric.theclinics.com

THE QUALITY ASSURANCE MOVEMENT

Most would accredit the Institute of Medicine for catalyzing the initial spark of interest in health care quality assurance. The organization's 1999 publication, *To Err is Human*, addressed the multitude of issues stemming from medical errors.[2] The effects of the study were sudden and drastic, drawing widespread attention to the problem from several directions and even influencing legislative change.

The appeal of reformation is deeply rooted in the prevention of avoidable patient injuries and deaths. Above all, it is these numbers that are and should be the most compelling fragments of data when it comes to the facilitation of quality improvement. However, the implications of a faulty medical system extend into all aspects of society, not the least of which are financial burdens. The study presented figures north of $17 billion in annual expenses as a result of medical errors. The health care system saw a dire decrease in trust, and physicians and patients alike suffered a loss of satisfaction and morale. The movement was, overall, one that would benefit the nation as a whole. In the same year, the Healthcare Research and Quality Act of 1999 was passed, promoting health care quality and improvement.

In *Crossing the Quality Chasm*, The Institute of Medicine described 6 attributes of quality in health care: safety, effectiveness, patient-family centeredness, timeliness, efficiency, and equity.[3] Several safety and quality efforts as well as hospital strategic plans have been built around those domains since that time. In 2003, The Agency for Healthcare Research and Quality (AHRQ) released a set of patient safety indicators (PSIs), to identify potentially adverse patient care events. After testing and validating the PSIs in adults, AHRQ revised them in 2006 and formulated a pediatric module. Subsequently, The Joint Commission's National Patient Safety Goals, AHRQ's PSIs, inpatient quality indicators, and Pediatric Quality Indicators were all released. The American Academy of Pediatrics (AAP) also came out with a statement summarizing information on how to develop and appropriately use quality measures to address issues that are relevant and important in pediatric health care.[4]

In 2012, 6 free-standing children's hospitals collectively developed a trigger tool using the Institute for Healthcare Improvement's adult-focused Global Trigger Tool model and pilot tested it to identify the most common causes of harm in pediatric inpatient settings. They found that harm to hospitalized children occurs at high rates, similar to all-cause harm in hospitalized adults.[5]

In 2007, the Centers for Medicare and Medicaid Services (CMS) announced its intent to use quality measures to guide reimbursement to hospitals. More recently, CMS also declared that state Medicaid programs could refuse to reimburse health care organizations for services rendered in treating certain provider-preventable conditions.

PEDIATRIC HOSPITAL MEDICINE AND INPATIENT HEALTH CARE

Pediatric hospital medicine (PHM) was formally recognized as a distinct discipline of pediatrics by AAP in 1999 when it approved the inception of Provisional Section on Hospital Care. The term "hospitalist," which is now a well-recognized designation, was originally coined by Wachter and Goldman in 1996.[6] A pediatric hospitalist is a pediatrician whose primary role is to take care of hospitalized patients and whose responsibilities also include patient care, teaching, mentoring, research, and leadership related to hospital medicine. The guiding principles for PHM programs are well delineated in AAP's policy statement released in October 2013.[7]

PHM is the fastest growing specialty of pediatrics.[8] Pediatric hospitalists possess the necessary skills to coordinate patient care, integrate hospital systems, and maximize efforts to enhance patient safety and influence positive outcomes in the complex inpatient environment. PHM groups are taking care of more patients, and are in charge of more processes in hospitals.[9] In addition to managing sick children with a multitude of medical and social problems, pediatric hospitalists are also faced with pressures to reduce length of stay, avoid hospital-acquired conditions, and prevent readmissions.

QUANTIFICATION

The clear first step toward being able to facilitate and track quality improvement lies in the formulation of measurable statistics. To see what is lacking, and thus see where progress can be made, a list of criteria needs to be determined. All gauges of patient safety and health care quality must be quantifiable. By coming to a consensus about these metrics, a systematic change can begin to be implemented, and improvements can be traced with concrete data.

To instigate this process, a strategic planning meeting was held in February of 2009, collectively by the Society of Hospital Medicine, the Section on Hospital Medicine of the AAP, and the Academic Pediatric Association, following which a Pediatric Hospital Medicine Dashboard Committee was formed that put together several consensus metrics and created a dashboard for PHM groups. This proposed dashboard was published in 2010.[10]

The goal of this dashboard was to promote internal and external monitoring and comparison among the various PHM groups, with the expectation that these will provide a starting point for data collection toward improving inpatient pediatric care. Metrics of this dashboard were separated into 6 categories: descriptive data, clinical quality data, nonclinical quality data, productivity measures, resource utilization, and group sustainability. Each category was then divided into 2 groups: "recommended metrics" and "metrics to consider."

Descriptive Data

Recommended metrics under this category include the following: Do hospitalists stay in-house overnight? How many clinical full-time equivalents (FTEs) are in the program? Are physician extenders used? Which areas do hospitalists cover? What are the total numbers of annual discharges? What is the payer mix? What are the top 10 diagnosis-related groups (DRGs)? What is the percentage of patients in each DRG? Metrics that are left for consideration by individual groups include the following: What is the case mix index for the hospitalist group? What percentage of patients are discharged in observation status? What percentage of patients are covered by resident teams, and so forth. Such descriptive data would allow for internal comparison within a single hospitalist group as well as comparison among local PHM groups, to facilitate more accurate benchmarking.

Clinical Quality Data

These can be either metrics that are required by reporting agencies, or evidence-based metrics or both. Length of stay (LOS) and The Joint Commission's core measures on asthma are the 2 recommended metrics under this category. Severity-adjusted LOS index, 15-day unplanned readmission rates, compliance with bronchiolitis guidelines, central line–associated blood stream infections (CLABSI), catheter-associated urinary tract infections (CAUTI), codes outside the intensive care unit, and hospital-acquired pressure ulcers are grouped under metrics to consider.

Nonclinical Quality Data

The 2 nonclinical quality metrics described under this category are patient satisfaction and referring physician satisfaction. These are likely to be more useful if done internally and compared year to year.

Productivity Measures Data

Metrics such as number of billable encounters per calendar day, relative value units (RVUs) per calendar day, RVUs per clinical FTE, distribution of evaluation/management (E/M) codes, and number of billed procedures per calendar day can be used to compare among similar types of groups, as well as for year-to-year internal comparisons by individual groups.

Resource Utilization Data

Average hospital charge per common DRG condition and opportunity days are metrics that can be used for discussions with the hospital administration to help show value. They are also useful for internal year-by-year comparisons for each group.

Group Sustainability Data

Metrics like hospitalist turnover, percentage of group attending PHM meeting, and number of hours worked per clinical FTE are helpful to assess overall stability and viability of a particular hospitalist group.

MEDICATION ERRORS IN HOSPITALIZED CHILDREN

Safely administering medications to hospitalized children is a complex task and requires several steps to be done correctly, to prevent medication errors. Medication dosing is more complicated in children because of the differences in their weight, body surface area, organ system maturity, and ability to metabolize and excrete drugs. Paucity of standardized dosing regimens for children also makes it more challenging. Additionally, several drugs are being used in children based on very limited evidence, without specific dosing guidelines or pediatric indications or formal approval from a US Food and Drug Administration licensing agency, putting children at increased risk of medication errors.[11]

Administration of medications may be associated with adverse reactions that are mostly unpredictable and nonpreventable, or adverse effects related to the inherent properties of the drug that are predictable but still nonpreventable. "Medication errors," on the other hand, often occur as a result of human mistakes or system failures and are, for the most part, preventable. An allergic reaction to a medication that happens to a patient with no history of drug allergy is considered an adverse reaction, but if the same reaction happens because of failure to obtain or document drug allergy, then it is considered a medication error. A medication error is defined as any preventable event that occurs during the process of ordering or delivering a medication, regardless of whether an injury occurred or the potential for injury was present.[12]

Errors can occur during medication selection, medication ordering, order transcription, drug formulation, drug dispensing, and drug administration. Medication errors can lead to patient discomfort, prolonged hospitalization, patient disability or death, increase in health care costs associated with hospitalization, increased medical liability for health care providers, and higher economic burden for the country.

The most commonly reported errors in both pediatric and adult patients are due to the following[13]:

- Wrong choice of medication
- Incorrect dosage
- Incorrect frequency of administration
- Wrong route of administration
- Delayed drug administration
- Failure to recognize drug interactions
- Failure to monitor for adverse effects
- Inadequate communication among the providers, patient, and family
- Inadequate system safeguards

MULTIDISCIPLINARY APPROACH TO REDUCE ERRORS

It is evident that errors are almost never the fault of an individual physician or health care worker. Treatment is a procedure that travels through multiple levels of responsibility. A chain of events is followed so as to accomplish every aspect of care. Any mistake made within 1 point in the chain can easily follow through the rest of the process. Hence, to begin improvements, a systematic approach must be adopted. Blaming a single provider will never lead to an improvement in quality, nor will quality-based statistics be impacted by any sort of fault-placing techniques. Resultantly, individuals in all fields, from prescribers to pharmacists, nurses, laboratory staff, and so forth, need to undergo particular self-checking methods. All links in the chain must be subject to certain responsibilities. The best course of action leading to a reduction in medical errors is one that systematically implements all of these responsibilities. Only then will we begin to see changes in quality of pediatric inpatient health care.[14]

This multidisciplinary tactic, when executed correctly, should stretch beyond the confines of the profession itself. Health care is a collaborative process, a mutual relationship. A small responsibility also must be placed on the patients themselves. The patients and families have an obligation to help prevent errors as well. Their awareness of drug allergies and health history, as well as the diligence to provide this information to the health care provider, are both components of a successful medical process. A shrewd family and patient will discuss questions and concerns with staff members and the staff should encourage such behavior to promote a symbiotic relationship among all members of the system. An optimized pediatric hospital structure lies in this amelioration of trust and understanding among the patients, their families, and health care providers. A systematic, multidisciplinary alteration and improvement plan is the single best course of action when it comes to ensuring higher quality in the field of PHM.

PROSPECTIVE METRICS FOR PEDIATRIC HOSPITAL MEDICINE

PHM's growth as a specialty is heavily dependent on developing and monitoring meaningful safety and quality metrics, which will reduce harm and improve inpatient child health outcomes. There are several prospective metrics that could be achievable targets for PHM. Even though they may lack validity, reliability, and feasibility, these metrics are high-impact, waste-reducing goals and worth pursuing as initial targets.[15]

CHILDREN'S HOSPITAL OF MICHIGAN'S SAFETY CULTURE

Despite the implementation of several different techniques by hospitals to improve their safety culture, serious safety events continue to occur nationwide. Safety events fall under 3 categories as defined by the Healthcare Performance Improvement

System[16] (HPIS): (1) near-miss event, does not reach the patient; (2) precursor event, reaches the patient but results in no harm or only minor temporary harm; and (3) serious safety event, reaches the patient and causes moderate to severe temporary harm, permanent harm, or death.

After analyzing what can be done, the potential benefits, and the obvious current pitfalls of the system that are in dire need of change, the Children's Hospital of Michigan (CHM), Detroit, has shifted its main focus toward promoting a safety culture by addressing safety events of all types.

CHM is a 125-year-old freestanding pediatric hospital with 228 beds, staffed by pediatric medical and surgical specialists. It is the only pediatric hospital within a large, 7-hospital medical system affiliated with The Wayne State University Medical School. CHM is a tertiary health center offering comprehensive medical and surgical care to children not only in the local community but also across the region and state.

Our safety initiative began with the formation of a hospital safety event team (HSET). Health care providers and ancillary staff were given training sessions on error recognition and prevention techniques. To promote a nonblame culture of error reporting, we started looking at "near-miss events" as opportunities for improvement and started celebrating them as "great catches." All reported events in our hospital get analyzed and brought to a close by the HSET. We also regularly evaluate provider-related safety events by peer review committee, and conduct a retrospective systems-based process review called root cause analysis to evaluate serious safety events.

INPATIENT SAFETY ROUNDING TOOL

At CHM, we have recently put together a checklist of inpatient items, which, we believe, if consistently used on rounds, has the potential to identify issues before they turn into problems. We call it "The Inpatient Safety Rounding Tool." Once implemented, we plan to assess the usefulness of this tool by conducting quality improvement studies (**Table 1**).

IMPROVING INPATIENT ASTHMA CARE AND PREVENTING ASTHMA READMISSIONS

We have incorporated an evidence-based, standardized, inpatient asthma care pathway in the electronic medical record as an easy-to-use power plan. For patients with asthma requiring pediatric intensive care unit (PICU) admission, asthma team consult is initiated while the patient is in the PICU, to enhance treatment efforts, reinforce asthma education, and help with discharge planning. Social work consult is also automatically obtained for such high-risk asthma patients, to support the family, and assist them with resources. Asthma Action Plan completion on discharge is monitored as a quality metric. Follow-up appointments with an asthma clinic are generally made before the patient is discharged from the hospital. Every attempt is made for high-risk patients with asthma to be seen in the asthma clinic within 2 weeks of discharge.

HAND HYGIENE MEASURES

As an initial step toward decreasing hospital-acquired infections, we started monitoring our adherence to hand washing in multiple hospital settings, including acute care units, emergency department, and operating rooms by deploying "secret shoppers." These hand hygiene compliance officers report their findings to the chief medical officer of CHM who in turn, shares the hand hygiene scores with all the staff on a monthly basis. This kind of intense monitoring with consistent feedback has raised our

Table 1
Inpatient safety rounding tool

#	Category	To Do During Rounds
1	Medication list	• Review medication doses • Check for medication interactions • Confirm if route of administration is appropriate • Change "scheduled meds" to "prn" when appropriate • Stop medications that are no longer required • Switch from parenteral to enteral alternatives when possible and appropriate • Reconcile medication at admission, transfer, and discharge • Update drug allergies
2	Diet	• Document all food allergies and restrictions • Note if patient is on a special diet (eg, ketogenic diet, modified Atkin diet, diabetic diet, gluten-free diet) • Specify what formula the patient is on, and the calories per ounce • Document the feeding route (eg, per oral, via gastric tube, gastro-jejunal tube, nasogastric tube) • Note if patient is an aspiration risk
3	Intravenous fluids	• Ensure appropriate rate and volume • Modify composition of fluids based on clinical indications and laboratory values • Stop intravenous fluids when no longer required
4	Peripheral intravenous lines	Examine intravenous site for leakage, swelling, pain, skin changes, and so forth
5	Central venous lines/peripherally inserted central catheter lines/ports	• Check for presence of these lines/devices • Check site for skin changes/discharge • Check if patient is spiking fevers
6	Gastric tube/gastro-jejunal tube/jejunal tube/nasogastric tube/nasojejunal tube	• Check for presence of these tubes • Note the exact type of tube • Note if the tube is being used • Confirm if formula and regimen correct
7	Decubitus ulcers	• Check for and document any skin breakdown/pressure ulcers in mobility-restricted patients • Place order for frequent position changes • Place order for appropriate bedding
8	Ventriculoperitoneal shunt/ventriculo-atrial shunt	• Check for presence of these devices • Look for symptoms/problems related to the device
9	Foley catheter	• Check for presence of urinary catheter • Verify the need for it • Remove if not needed

(*continued on next page*)

Table 1 (continued)	
# Category	**To Do During Rounds**
10 Venous thrombo-embolism	• Check if patient is at risk • Consider sequential compression device • Ambulate as soon as possible • Consider heparin prophylaxis
11 Vaccines and newborn screen	• Check Michigan Care Improvement Registry for vaccination status and newborn screen report • Consider ordering influenza and/or other missing vaccines as appropriate
12 Discharge planning	• Ensure follow-up appointments with primary care provider and specialist clinics • Check need for prior-authorization of medication • Check insurance status, transportation needs • Consider social work consult as appropriate • Anticipate and order durable medical equipment and other home-care needs

institution's hand hygiene scores from less than 85% to more than 96% in the past 4 years.

OTHER METRICS

CHM's safety goals also include practicing standardized hand-off communication; completing medication reconciliation on admission, transfers, and discharge; eliminating subcutaneous infiltration of intravenous fluids; reducing hospital-acquired pressure ulcers; and preventing CLABSIs and CAUTIs. As we track our progress and keep records of the data we collect, CHM hopes that our quality assurance (QA) mechanisms result in a significant reduction in lives lost and injuries caused by medical errors.

SUMMARY

Developing an efficient process that will reliably detect medical errors is key to advancing safety in hospitalized pediatric patients. Multi-institutional networking studies have shown that using quality improvement (QI) methods and implementing best practices can achieve improved results.[17] Encouraging QI methods, following safety principles, effectively using information technology, developing standardized protocols, and implementing best practices are some of the ways by which health care organizations can successfully reduce harm to patients and also reduce resource utilization.

The QA movement is a collective drive for continual improvement. The fundamental aspiration of the health care system, and of all those involved in it, is a desire to provide outstanding patient care. This mindset is shared by all medical professionals, and is the basis of the improvement we strive for. As a result, the field has a perpetual willingness to adapt. To satisfy the growing need for increased health care quality, this imperfect system must use this ambitious attitude to achieve superior quality. The proposed metrics serve as a tangible aspiration to help facilitate this. The process itself is composed of nothing new; QA is simply a system of checks on our work. An addition as simple as this one with the capacity to yield just drastic results cannot be ignored, especially when it comes to the health and safety of children.

REFERENCES

1. Kaushal R, Bates DW, Landrigan C, et al. Medication errors and adverse drug events in pediatric inpatients. JAMA 2001;285(16):2114–20.
2. National Research Council. To err is human: building a safer health system. Washington, DC: The National Academies Press; 2000.
3. Institute of Medicine. Crossing the quality chasm. A new health system for the 21st century. Washington, DC: National Academy Press; 2001.
4. Hodgson ES, Simpson L, Lannon CM. Principles for the development and use of quality measures. Pediatrics 2008;121(2):411–8.
5. Stockwell DC, Bisarya H, Classen DC, et al. A trigger tool to detect harm in pediatric inpatient settings. Pediatrics 2015;135:1036–42.
6. Wachter RM, Goldman L. The emerging role of "hospitalists" in the American health care system. N Engl J Med 1996;335(7):514–7.
7. Section on Hospital Medicine. Guiding principles for pediatric hospital medicine programs. Pediatrics 2013;132(4):782–6.
8. Friedman J. The hospitalist movement in general pediatrics. Curr Opin Pediatr 2010;22(6):785–90.
9. Freed GL, Dunham KM, Research advisory committee of the American board of pediatrics. Pediatric hospitalists: training, current practice, and career goals. J Hosp Med 2009;4(3):179–86.
10. Hain PD, Daru J, Robbins E, et al. A proposed dashboard for pediatric hospital medicine groups. Hosp Pediatr 2012;2(2):59–70.
11. D'Antonio YC, Cohen MR. Pediatric medication errors. In: Cohen MR, editor. Medication errors. Washington, DC: American Pharmaceutical Association; 1999. p. 16.1–8.
12. Joint Commission on Accreditation of Healthcare Organizations. 2002 hospital accreditation standards. Oakbrook Terrace (IL): Joint Commission on Accreditation of Healthcare Organizations; 2002. p. 51–61, 101, 111–115, 148, 161–174, 345.
13. Crowley E, Williams R, Cousins D. Medication errors in children: a descriptive summary of medication error reports submitted to the United States Pharmacopeia. Curr Ther Res 2001;26:627–40.
14. Stucky ER. Prevention of medication errors in the pediatric inpatient setting. Pediatrics 2003;112(2):431–6.
15. Shen MW, Percelay J. Quality measures in pediatric hospital medicine: moneyball or looking for Fabio? Hosp Pediatr 2012;2:121.
16. Throop C, Stockmeier C. The HPI SEC & SSER patient safety measurement system for healthcare. Virginia: HPI White Paper Series; 2009.
17. Billett AL, Colletti RB, Mandel KE, et al. Exemplar pediatric collaborative improvement networks: achieving results. Pediatrics 2013;131(Suppl 4):S196–203.

Advanced Technology in Pediatric Intensive Care Units: Have They Improved Outcomes?

Sean A. Frederick, MD

KEYWORDS

- Pediatric • Intensive care • Outcome • Electronic health record/EHR
- Medical informatics • Computerized provider order entry/CPOE
- Clinical decision support/CDS

KEY POINTS

- In medicine, providers strive to produce quality outcomes and work to continually improve those outcomes.
- Whether it is reducing cost, decreasing length of stay, mitigating nosocomial infections, or improving survival, there are a myriad of complex factors that contribute to each outcome.
- One of the greatest challenges to outcome improvement is in pediatric intensive care units, which tend to host the sickest, most complex, smallest, and frailest of pediatric patients.

INTRODUCTION

An outcome is something that follows as a result of an act or an intervention; the outcome may either be positive or negative. In medicine, providers strive to produce quality outcomes and work to continually improve those outcomes. Whether it is reducing cost, decreasing length of stay, mitigating nosocomial infections, or improving survival, there are a myriad of complex factors that contribute to each outcome. One of the greatest challenges to outcome improvement is in pediatric intensive care units (ICUs), which tend to host the sickest, most complex, smallest, and frailest pediatric patients.

Compared with medicine, the advent of the various subspecialists in pediatric intensive care is recent. For example, The Society of Critical Care Medicine (SCCM), representing the adult intensive care community, recognized pediatric critical care as a discrete field, and created the section of pediatric critical care within the SCCM in

Disclosure: The author has nothing to disclose.
University of Pittsburgh Medical Center Newborn Medicine Program, 300 Halket Street, Pittsburgh, PA 15213, USA
E-mail address: fredericksa@upmc.edu

1981.[1,2] A sub-board in critical care medicine was established by the American Board of Pediatrics and the first certifying examination was offered in 1987.[1,2] Neonatology has been present slightly longer, with the terms neonatology and neonatologist first introduced in 1960.[3] In 1975, the first examination of the Sub-Board of Neonatal-Perinatal Medicine of the American Board of Pediatrics and the first meeting of the Perinatal Section of the American Academy of Pediatrics were held.[3]

Despite being young, these fields have benefited tremendously from advances in medical knowledge and technologies to not only help improve day-to-day patient care but to improve outcomes as well. One of the greatest nonmedical advances in the past several decades that has changed daily patient care practices has been the introduction of the electronic medical record (EMR) and with it medical informatics. This change that has occurred in the medical work environment has the potential to facilitate communication and enforce adherence of global best practices.[4]

Computerization has been a hallmark of the twenty-first century, with every major industry investing heavily in these technologies to reduce cost, increase efficiencies, and improve outcomes; health care is no exception to this growing trend. After decades of technological laggard, medicine has begun to acclimatize to the digital data age.[5] The Health Information Technology for Economic and Clinical Health (HITECH) Act of 2009, which was signed into law, represents the largest US initiative to date that is designed to encourage widespread use of electronic health records.[6] EMR systems can include many potential capabilities, but 3 particular functionalities hold great promise in improving the quality of care and reducing costs at the health care system level: clinical decision support (CDS) tools, computerized physician order entry (CPOE) systems, and health information exchange (HIE).[6] In the ever-changing world of health care delivery these basic EMR functionalities form the basis for improving quality of care and reducing costs; two key health care–related outcomes that are being benchmarked against respective peer groups.

Also, a technology that is increasingly being adopted is telemedicine service. Many institutions are using ICU-based telemedicine services for remote monitoring, staffing, and/or consultation to aid in outcome improvements. Simply stated, ICU telemedicine uses audiovisual technology to provide critical care services from a remote location.[7,8] In its most common form, ICU telemedicine consists of remote monitoring of ICU patients using fixed installations, either continuously or during nighttime hours.[8,9] Telemedicine can potentially improve ICU outcomes by increasing access to the expertise of dedicated intensivist physicians,[8,10] facilitating early recognition of physiologic deterioration,[8,11] and prompting bedside providers to implement routine evidence-based practices.[8,12]

ELECTRONIC MEDICAL RECORDS

EMRs have become central to modern medicine. The HITECH Act of 2009 has thrust EMRs into the forefront of every health care organization's agenda. In addition to the federal mandates associated with the HITECH Act, several factors have influenced the adoption of EMRs; these factors include, but are not limited to, supporting patient care activities, cost cutting and operational efficiencies, big-data analysis of patient health records, and incentive dollars associated with meaningful use. The power of EMRs is only matched by their complexities. EMRs vary from home-grown systems in single organizations with the necessary technical and managerial capacity; to interoperability standards for linking multiple information technology systems; to top-down, government-driven, national implementations of standardized, commercial software applications.[13] However varied the systems remain, they share a common goal: to create a single longitudinal record for each patient that can be digitally shared and accessed by different health care providers to create a cohesive and safer patient care experience.

COMPUTERIZED PROVIDER ORDER ENTRY AND CLINICAL DECISION SUPPORT

Implementation of an EMR system with CPOE and/or CDS can provide an important foundation for decreasing medication errors and harm.[14–17]

Computerized Provider Order Entry

CPOE systems provide the ability to enter orders for patients into a computer, allowing electronic transmission of the orders to the appropriate department (eg, pharmacy, radiology, and laboratory).[18] CPOE is the feature of EMR implementation that arguably offers the greatest quality and patient safety benefits.[19] However, CPOE adoption, success, and outcome improvement are often heavily influenced by local factors.

Studies have shown both positive and negative outcomes associated with the introduction of EMR CPOE systems. Longhurst and colleagues[20] showed a decrease in hospital-wide mortality following CPOE implementation at Lucile Packard Children's Hospital at Stanford, contrasting an earlier study published in 2006 by Han and colleagues,[21] which observed an unexpected increase in mortality coincident with CPOE implementation in a pediatric ICU. The hospitals in these two contrasting studies used the same EMR software vendor, suggesting that local implementation decisions are a critical factor in determining the safety performance of CPOE systems.[17]

Clinical Decision Support

Decision support tools have been used by the medical profession for decades and evolved with technology to become largely computer based and widely accessible to all clinicians.[22] CDS often refers to electronic suggestions or reminders linked to a patient's electronic data and integrated within a clinician's workflow, and provides much of the value in implementing CPOE systems.[19] CDS tools can be implemented to influence a variety of factors that directly affect patient care outcomes. Among the most important CDS tools used in pediatrics are those centered around medication ordering and administration, such as drug-drug interactions; allergy alerts; clinical condition correlation (eg, medications that need to have altered doses related to clinical conditions); and, key in pediatrics, dose range checking. Accurate and informed prescribing is essential to ensure the safe and effective use of medications in pediatric patients.[23]

In addition to medication ordering and administration, CDS tools have evolved to include antibiotic stewardship,[24] vaccination administrations and reminders,[25] prediction tools,[22] and suggestions for therapeutic interventions,[26] but these are just a few of the possibilities; however, because comprehensive CDS tools are not standard in EMR systems, their implementation is often limited by local factors, such as cost, time, and resource allocation.

TELEMEDICINE AND REMOTE INTENSIVE CARE UNIT MONITORING

ICU service is an important and often expensive competent of hospital care. ICUs are responsible for caring for the sickest patients in the hospital on any given day and are staffed by highly specialized and well-trained individuals. However, because of various constraints it is not always possible to staff ICUs around the clock, 7 days a week, 365 days a year. It has been estimated that approximately 1% of the US gross domestic product is consumed in the care of ICU patients.[10,27] Despite this considerable investment of resources, there is wide variation in ICU organization[28,29] and studies have suggested that differences in ICU organization may affect patient outcome.[10] Given the complexity associated with adequately staffing ICUs, technology has become an increasing focus to provide adequate staffing power, knowledge base, and monitoring of patient care. ICU telemedicine is a novel approach for providing critical care services from a distance.[8]

Comprehensive ICU telemedicine programs that provide continuous patient monitoring by an off-site team of critical care professionals have the ability to recognize physiologic instability and to render care that is timely and triggered by patient factors.[9] Telemedicine can potentially improve ICU outcomes by increasing access to the expertise of dedicated intensivist physicians.[8,10] This approach may be preferable where staffing is inadequate because of various constraints. In addition, institutions with less case/clinical experience may rely on centers of excellence in facilitating care, allowing patients to stay regionally when feasible, while still providing the highest level of care and monitoring. These benefits are often stated, but literature is scant on reporting and showing clear benefit. Studies of the practice of ICU telemedicine are limited in part by the lack of reliable and practical methods for measurement of ICU and ICU telemedicine program structural and process elements[9]; however, there is some accumulating evidence that ICU telemedicine may be associated with decreases in mortality and hospital length of stay, as well as improved adherence to consequential best practices and lower rates of preventable complications.[30]

DATA TRENDING AND REVIEW

The EMR has become a powerful tool for data collection because of its ease and ability to store vast amounts of real-time clinical data. The amount of clinical information that providers encounter daily creates an environment for information overload.[31] The potential dangers underlying this information overload relate to the inability of practitioners to distinguish pertinent from irrelevant information.[31,32] In general, the potential for information overload has been handled well and the benefits have been readily apparent; most institutions have shown improved outcomes, increased productivity, and fewer errors associated with EMR use.[20,31,33–36]

BIG DATA AND PREDICTIVE ANALYTICS

EMRs generate massive amounts of data, commonly referred to as big data, that are difficult to interpret via traditional software analytics. These data, on the scale of terabytes and larger, hold key pieces of information vital to the health care functions surrounding management and outcomes. The identification of high-value data presents a significant challenge to any health care provider.[37] The promise of supporting a wide range of medical and health care functions, including CDS, disease surveillance, and population health management,[38–42] is what many organizations are investing and relying heavily on for the future.

Big data in health care is overwhelming not only because of its volume but also because of the diversity of data types and the speed at which it must be managed.[42,43] Managing big data is key, because it has the potential to significantly influence modern medicine. The hope is for improved outcomes, reduced cost, predictive preventive care, enhanced clinical effectiveness guidelines, and greater targeted research. Big data analytics and adaption also spur greater patient engagement and enhanced targeted population health management tools.

Application and interpretation of big data in the ICU is an important focus to try to improve outcomes and the quality of care, because this may be the difference between life and death. Such tools as early warning systems are paramount and often standard practice to aid clinicians in identifying a potential impending critical situation or patient decompensation. These systems were designed to be frequently used and simple hand-scored calculations based on a composite of limited data points, often centered on patient vital signs. Systems such as Modified Early Warning Score[44] and Pediatric Early Warning System[45] that were useful in their applications are being challenged by newer systems, such as the Rothman index, which are able to calculate and recalculate scores on a minute-by-minute basis as new data are acquired. Such (newer) systems could deliver timely, accurate, longitudinally trended acuity information that could aid in earlier detection of declining patient condition as well as improving sensitivity and specificity of early warning systems alarms.[46]

OUTCOMES

Daily work in the ICU involves multitasking and responding to unpredictable events, such as patient changes in status and work flow interruptions. These features combine to produce an environment in which providers must rely on implicit knowledge and internal task management schema to guide the prioritization and performance of tasks.[4] The unpredictable nature of the workload, patient volume, daily tasks, and emergencies is challenging in this environment, which in turn may make the goal of improving outcomes equally challenging. Healthcare outcomes are central to the delivery of quality medical care; with a growing focus on value-based care, being able to measure and improve outcomes is paramount to showing effectiveness.

Multidisciplinary teams of ICU providers make decisions and deliver care to acutely ill patients in complex environments. The interaction between providers and technology in these environments may have a profound impact on the quality of care delivered to the patient.[4] Improving outcomes in the ICU relies on a combination of human factors, complex medical knowledge, unpredictable events, and vast amounts of data interpretation and review. Because of the broad scope of how health care is delivered in the United States and across the world, each institution should design interventions that are scaled to their culture and health care delivery structure to best improve their desired outcomes; to date, there is no one-size-fits-all model.

SUMMARY

The landscape of modern medicine continues to change and evolve. During the last century, rapid advancements in medical technology and subspecialty care have transformed acute care hospitals into highly complex institutions offering a wide variety of medical and surgical interventions.[4] The EMR is now an expected standard and vital for day-to-day operations of many institutions, including ICUs; EMRs have become common in many large tertiary referral centers. For the many institutions that have converted to this digital environment, a day without an EMR would be unthinkable. As EMRs become more prevalent, their potential impact on quality and safety, both negative and positive, will be increased.[37] For decades it has been well known that human factors are implicated in most medical errors[47] and, despite all of medicine's advances, the 1 component in the equation of care delivery that does not change is the human factor. The interaction between providers and technology in these environments may have a profound impact on the quality of care delivered to patients (**Fig. 1**).[4]

The adoption of EMR has been proposed as being valuable for driving improvements in the quality of that care[4]; however, adoption of EMRs in itself does not equal

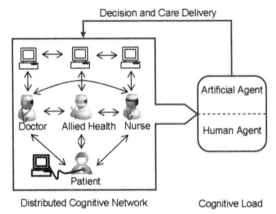

Fig. 1. The distributed cognitive network; understanding how multidisciplinary teams deliver care in complex environments. A network of providers, using a variety of environmental artifacts (data from EMRs, bedside monitors, to-do lists from other providers, notes taken on rounds) make decisions and act on them to deliver care to the patients. Understanding how that network functions, where its vulnerabilities lie, and how it reacts to changes in the operational environment facilitates the emergence of tools (organizational, decision support, smart alerts, novel user interfaces, and ambient intelligence applications) that improve the reliability, efficacy, and safety of the care delivered to the bedside. The artificial agents (eg, health information technology–enabled decision supports) act in cooperation with the human agents (nurses, doctors) to facilitate the development of a care plan. (*From* Pickering BW, Litell JM, Herasevich V, et al. Clinical review: the hospital of the future - building intelligent environments to facilitate safe and effective acute care delivery. Crit Care 2012;16(2):220; with permission.)

improved quality of care or outcomes. For example, in order to provide safe and effective critical care, bedside providers need to have an accurate mental model of the patient; a clear picture in their heads of the patient's background, physiology, and potential response to therapies or interventions.[4] Although this mental model is something that the EMR may assist in synthesizing, it cannot perform the task completely because there are key human-performed factors that are used in creating a plan of care; in the ICU these human factors may occur in isolation or as part of a complex multidisciplinary team. There are a myriad of factors in the ICU that vary from hospital to hospital/unit to unit and that influence this as well. Local institutional factors may play the most important role in improving outcomes and making the delivery of care safer.

REFERENCES

1. Epstein D, Brill JE. A history of pediatric critical care medicine. Pediatr Res 2005; 58:987–96.
2. Downes JJ. The historical evolution, current status, and prospective development of pediatric critical care. Crit Care Clin 1992;8(1):1–22.
3. Philip AG. The evolution of neonatology. Pediatr Res 2005;58(4):799–815.
4. Pickering BW, Litell JM, Herasevich V, et al. Clinical review: The hospital of the future - building intelligent environments to facilitate safe and effective acute care delivery. Crit Care 2012;16(2):220.
5. Belle A, Thiagarajan R, Soroushmehr SMR, et al. Big data analytics in healthcare. Biomed Res Int 2015;2015:370194.

6. Menachemi N, Collum TH. Benefits and drawbacks of electronic health record systems. Risk Manag Healthc Policy 2011;4:47–55.
7. Garland A, Gershengorn HB. Staffing in ICUs: physicians and alternative staffing models. Chest 2013;143(1):214–21.
8. Kahn JM, Cicero BD, Wallace DJ, et al. Adoption of intensive care unit telemedicine in the United States. Crit Care Med 2014;42(2):362–8.
9. Lilly CM, Fisher KA, Ries M, et al. A national ICU telemedicine survey: validation and results. Chest 2012;142(1):40–7.
10. Pronovost PJ, Angus DC, Dorman T, et al. Physician staffing patterns and clinical outcomes in critically ill patients: a systematic review. JAMA 2002;288(17): 2151–62.
11. Siebig S, Kuhls S, Imhoff M, et al. Collection of annotated data in a clinical validation study for alarm algorithms in intensive care–a methodologic framework. J Crit Care 2010;25(1):128–35.
12. Weiss CH, Moazed F, McEvoy CA, et al. Prompting physicians to address a daily checklist and process of care and clinical outcomes: a single-site study. Am J Respir Crit Care Med 2011;184(6):680–6.
13. Robertson A, Cresswell K, Takian A, et al. Implementation and adoption of nationwide electronic health records in secondary care in England: qualitative analysis of interim results from a prospective national evaluation. BMJ 2010; 341:c4564.
14. Kaushal R, Shojania KG, Bates DW. Effects of computerized physician order entry and clinical decision support systems on medication safety: a systematic review. Arch Intern Med 2003;163(12):1409–16.
15. Kuperman GJ, Bobb A, Payne TH, et al. Medication-related clinical decision support in computerized provider order entry systems: a review. J Am Med Inform Assoc 2007;14(1):29–40.
16. Upperman JS, Staley P, Friend K, et al. The impact of hospitalwide computerized physician order entry on medical errors in a pediatric hospital. J Pediatr Surg 2005;40(1):57–9.
17. Longhurst CA, Palma JP, Grisim LM, et al. Using an evidence-based approach to EMR implementation to optimize outcomes and avoid unintended consequences. J Healthc Inf Manag 2013;27(3):79–83.
18. Lehmann CU, Kim GR. Computerized provider order entry and patient safety. Pediatr Clin North Am 2006;53(6):1169–84.
19. Palma JP, Sharek PJ, Classen DC, et al. Neonatal informatics: computerized physician order entry. Neoreviews 2011;12:393–6.
20. Longhurst CA, Parast L, Sandborg CI, et al. Decrease in hospital-wide mortality rate after implementation of a commercially sold computerized physician order entry system. Pediatrics 2010;126(1):14–21.
21. Han YY, Carcillo JA, Venkataraman ST, et al. Unexpected increased mortality after implementation of a commercially sold computerized physician order entry system. Pediatrics 2005;116(6):1506–12.
22. Williams CN, Bratton SL, Hirshberg EL. Computerized decision support in adult and pediatric critical care. World J Crit Care Med 2013;2(4):21–8.
23. Stultz JS, Nahata MC. Computerized clinical decision support for medication prescribing and utilization in pediatrics. J Am Med Inform Assoc 2012;19(6): 942–53.
24. Hum RS, Cato K, Sheehan B, et al. Developing clinical decision support within a commercial electronic health record system to improve antimicrobial prescribing in the neonatal ICU. Appl Clin Inform 2014;5(2):368–87.

25. Stockwell MS, Fiks AG. Utilizing health information technology to improve vaccine communication and coverage. Hum Vaccin Immunother 2013;9(8): 1802–11.
26. Timbie JW, Damberg CL, Schneider EC, et al. A conceptual framework and protocol for defining clinical decision support objectives applicable to medical specialties. BMC Med Inform Decis Mak 2012;12:93.
27. Halpern NA, Bettes L, Greenstein R. Federal and nationwide intensive care units and healthcare costs: 1986-1992. Crit Care Med 1994;22:2001–7.
28. Pronovost PJ, Jencks M, Dorman T, et al. Organizational characteristics of intensive care units related to outcomes of abdominal aortic surgery. JAMA 1999;281: 1310–2.
29. Groeger JS, Strosberg MA, Halpern NA, et al. Descriptive analysis of critical care units in the United States. Crit Care Med 1992;20:846–63.
30. Lilly CM, Cody S, Zhao H, et al. Hospital mortality, length of stay, and preventable complications among critically ill patients before and after tele-ICU reengineering of critical care processes. JAMA 2011;16:2175–83.
31. Ellsworth MA, Lang TR, Pickering BW, et al. Clinical data needs in the neonatal intensive care unit electronic medical record. BMC Med Inform Decis Mak 2014;14:92.
32. Potter AK, Johnson DP. Extracting the pertinent from the irrelevant. Minn Med 1994;77(4):58.
33. Ahmed A, Chandra S, Herasevich V, et al. The effect of two different electronic health record user interfaces on intensive care provider task load, errors of cognition, and performance. Crit Care Med 2011;39(7):1626–34.
34. Bates DW. Using information technology to reduce rates of medication errors in hospitals. BMJ 2000;320(7237):788–91.
35. Bates DW, Leape LL, Cullen DJ, et al. Effect of computerized physician order entry and a team intervention on prevention of serious medication errors. JAMA 1998;280(15):1311–6.
36. Palma JP, Sharek PJ, Longhurst CA. Impact of electronic medical record integration of a handoff tool on sign-out in a newborn intensive care unit. J Perinatol 2011;31(5):311–7.
37. Pickering BW, Herasevich V, Ahmed A, et al. Novel representation of clinical information in the ICU. Appl Clin Inform 2010;1(2):116–31.
38. Burghard C. Big data and analytics key to accountable care success. IDC Health Insights; 2012.
39. Dembosky A. Data prescription for better healthcare. Financial Times; 2012. Available at: http://www.ft.com/intl/cms/s/2/55cbca5a-4333-11e2-aa8f-00144fe abdc0.html.
40. Feldman B, Martin EM, Skotnes T. Big data in health care hype and hope. Dr Bonnie 360; 2012. Available at: https://www.ghdonline.org/uploads/big-data-in-healthcare_B_Kaplan_2012.pdf.
41. Fernandes L, O'Connor M, Weaver V. Big data, bigger outcomes: healthcare is embracing the big data movement, hoping to revolutionize HIM by distilling vast collection of data for specific analysis. J AHIMA 2012;83(10):38–42.
42. Raghupathi W, Raghupathi V. Big data analytics in healthcare: promise and potential. Health Inf Sci Syst 2014;2:3.
43. Frost, Sullivan. Drowning in big data? Reducing information technology complexities and costs for healthcare organizations. Available at: http://www.emc.com/collateral/analyst-reports/frost-sullivan-reducing-information-technology-complexities-ar.pdf. Accessed August, 2015.

44. Subbe CP, Kruger M, Rutherford P, et al. Validation of a modified early warning score in medical admissions. QJM 2001;94:521–6.
45. Duncan H, Hutchison J, Parshuram CS. The Pediatric Early Warning System Score: a severity of illness score to predict urgent medical need in hospitalized children. J Crit Care 2006;21(3):271–8.
46. Finlay GD, Rothman MJ, Smith RA. Measuring the modified early warning score and the Rothman Index: advantages of utilizing the electronic medical record in an early warning system. J Hosp Med 2014;9(2):116–9.
47. Cooper JB, Newbower RS, Long CD, et al. Preventable anesthesia mishaps: a study of human factors. Anesthesiology 1978;16:399–406.

ABCs of Safety and Quality for the Pediatric Resident and Fellow

Emily Mathias, MD, Usha Sethuraman, MD*

KEYWORDS

- Quality improvement • Patient safety • Graduate medical education
- Next accreditation system • Clinical learning environment review

KEY POINTS

- As part of their Next Accreditation System, the Accreditation Council for Graduate Medical Education set forth expectations for trainee proficiency in health care quality and patient safety.
- The Clinical Learning Environment Review was established with the primary goals of learning how to best optimize patient safety and clinical quality where trainees are providing care.
- Teaching the basic principles of patient safety and quality improvement methodology can be accomplished through didactic sessions, but incorporating quality improvement projects into the curriculum has been shown to further engage learners and help facilitate development of application skills.

INTRODUCTION

All the flowers of all the tomorrows are in the seeds of today

—Indian proverb

The US health care system is plagued by unnecessary variations in care resulting in many children receiving suboptimal health care. With the publication of *To Err is Human* and *Crossing the Quality Chasm*, the Institute of Medicine brought to light the shortcomings of our health care system in providing safe, high-quality health care for patients. The call for a national effort to address these shortcomings has resulted in a surge of support for focused initiatives aimed at eliminating disparities in health care delivery and improving safety in health care. It is now recognized that

Disclosures: None.
Pediatric Emergency Medicine, Carman and Ann Adams Department of Pediatrics, Wayne State University, 3901 Beaubien Boulevard, Detroit, MI 48201, USA
* Corresponding author.
E-mail address: USethura@dmc.org

Pediatr Clin N Am 63 (2016) 303–315
http://dx.doi.org/10.1016/j.pcl.2015.11.003
0031-3955/16/$ – see front matter © 2016 Elsevier Inc. All rights reserved.

improving the overall health care system requires physicians with competence in safety and quality improvement (QI) skills.

Despite the growing popularity of this movement, there remain barriers to progress.[1] Although recognizing specific problems and providing targeted solutions have provided some amount of measurable benefit, it has become apparent that the primary obstacle to change lies in the culture of medicine itself,[1] a culture that, in its not-so-distant past, was deeply committed to the ideals of autonomy, authority, and self-reliance—all of which have been shown to detract from an environment focused on achieving safety.

With this in mind, there has been a push toward a grassroots effort to start promoting safety and QI early on within the course of medical education. By teaching core concepts of quality care and patient safety to young physicians, a generation of health care professionals capable of passing on these values to their colleagues and, most importantly, future trainees becomes a reality. Hence, there is a growing impetus to incorporate patient safety and QI into the educational framework of physicians in training.

PATIENT SAFETY AND QUALITY IMPROVEMENT AS PART OF GRADUATE MEDICAL EDUCATION

The need for engagement and integration of QI and patient safety initiatives within graduate medical education (GME) was realized early on.[2] Residents and fellows make up a significant number of the providers involved in patient interactions within academic medical institutions. Recognizing their unique position on the front lines of care, their role in patient-centered improvement processes becomes critical to a health care system's success. It has been suggested that a coordinated approach is required to train residents in QI and safety issues. Repeated exposure to QI and performing mentored projects and application during residency years facilitate enhanced training. However, most QI training still occurs in the form of lectures, modules that are self-guided, and electives. In a recent survey of graduating residents, QI practice was noted as the biggest deficiency of training programs, highlighting the existing holes in this aspect of training and the urgent need for improvement. Specifically, efforts to involve residents in local or institutional QI efforts seem to be poor, resulting in missed opportunities for training. This point is important to note, especially because institutional commitment to involving residents in QI is associated with a higher rate of resident participation.

As part of their Next Accreditation System (NAS), the Accreditation Council for Graduate Medical Education (ACGME) set forth expectations for trainee proficiency in health care quality and patient safety.[3] Of the 6 core competencies outlined by the NAS, practice-based learning and improvement (PBLI) and systems-based practice (SBP) domains mandate that residents and fellows be assessed on their ability to enhance the quality of care and advocate for patient safety.[4] Subcompetencies within these core domains further define developmental milestones relating to QI and patient safety (**Box 1**).[5]

"*Coordinate patient care within the health system relevant to their clinical specialty.*" This subcompetency is focused on developing trainees' ability to assist patients and their families in navigating the complex health care system.[6] The progression through the milestone highlights open communication and collaboration between care teams; seamless transition of care between settings, including written care plans; and recognition of possible barriers to patients and families in achieving coordinated health care. All of these aspects of care are centered on the concept of a *medical home*, the model of care delivery advocated by the American Academy of Pediatrics (AAP).[7]

Box 1

General pediatrics reporting milestones: QI- and patient safety–related competencies

Core Competency Domain	Reporting Milestone Subcompetency	Description
SBP	SBP1	Coordinate patient care within the health care system relevant to their clinical specialty.
	SBP2	Advocate for quality patient care and optimal patient care systems.
	SBP3	Work in interprofessional teams to enhance patient safety and improve patient care quality.
PBLI	PBLI3	Systematically analyze practice using QI methods, and implement changes with the goal of practice improvement.

Adapted from Accreditation Council for Graduate Medical Education. Pediatric Milestones Project. 2013. Available at: https://www.acgme.org/acgmeweb/Portals/0/PDFs/Milestones/320_PedsMilestonesProject.pdf. Accessed August 2, 2015.

The medical home is defined by the AAP as one that is accessible, continuous, family centered, coordinated, compassionate, and culturally effective.[7] This patient-centered model facilitates in providing high-quality, safe patient and family experiences, and improves health care outcomes. This point is highlighted by the example of a patient with chronic medical problems, such as ventilator-dependent respiratory disease, seizures, hydrocephalus, and feeding problems requiring G tube feeds. Such a patient is best benefitted by a multidisciplinary team approach, addressing all aspects of the child's care with the primary care team.

"Advocate for quality patient care and optimal patient care systems." This subcompetency is centered on the idea of the physician advocate.[6] In progressing through their training, physicians should develop skills and knowledge that enable them to address concerns of groups, ultimately improving the quality of a system. At the highest level of achievement, trainees should be an active participant in the QI and patient safety initiatives of their health care system and demonstrate an eagerness to make an impact in the community. An example would be involvement in a project disseminating information to the community about bicycle safety and helmet use.

"Work in interprofessional teams to enhance patient safety and improve patient care quality." This subcompetency hones in on the importance of multidisciplinary teamwork in providing optimal quality of care and a safe patient environment.[6] Physicians in training must strive to use the full professional capabilities of all team members, practicing within the scope of their discipline. By understanding the complementary nature of an interprofessional environment, they become excellent team members, team leaders, and role models for others.

"Systematically analyze practice using quality improvement methods, and implement changes with the goal of practice improvement." Physicians in training progress through this subcompetency by developing the knowledge, skills, and attitudes needed to systematically analyze practice using the standards of medical care, change management principles, and QI methodology.[6] It is understood that the degree to which trainees progress through this milestone depends on the clinical environment. With this in mind, advancement is achieved by thinking and acting systemically as well as demonstrating insight into how improvement opportunities can be applied on a larger scale. For example, if there is an identified variation in timing of the first dose of steroids given for children with an asthma exacerbation in the emergency department, a resident or fellow in training may be involved in a mentored quality

assessment and improvement project that addresses this deficiency with the ultimate aim of improving care of children with asthma exacerbation.

The Pediatric Milestone Project does address that achieving these competencies can be particularly challenging given some of the barriers that exist within the current system.[6] For example, the time-limited rotations/blocks that are the current model for a resident's schedule makes is difficult to foster team relationships. Additionally, the QI and patient safety movements are relatively new areas of focus within the medical community; some academic training institutions have yet to fully develop focused initiatives and programs. Therefore, trainees' exposure to a culture that promotes interdependent functioning is highly variable. Given the potential obstacles, the ACGME developed a complementary program along with the NAS in order to promote a learning environment that upholds the principles paramount to quality and safety.

THE CLINICAL LEARNING ENVIRONMENT: THE FOUNDATION OF QUALITY IMPROVEMENT IN MEDICAL EDUCATION

The Clinical Learning Environment Review (CLER) program sets forth the "expectations for an optimal clinical learning environment to achieve safe and high quality patient care."[8] It was established with the primary goals of learning how to best optimize patient safety and clinical quality where trainees are providing care and how to best prepare trainees to meet the needs of an evolving health care system.[8] As a key component of the NAS, CLER was designed to assess ACGME-accredited institutional efforts to incorporate quality and safety training into their curriculum engaging their trainees in the 6 important areas of health care quality and patient safety along with feedback on how they can improve the process. The CLER program provides ongoing site visits by an expert committee who assess the clinical learning environment, explain expectations, and share opportunities for improvement.[8] As the purpose of these visits is intended to be formative, information gathered is being tracked and analyzed but currently has no impact on institutional accreditation.[8] Aggregated information from site visits, along with emerging research, are used to optimize the program.

The 6 focus areas of CLER performance evaluation include patient safety, QI, care transitions, supervision, duty hours and fatigue management and mitigation, and professionalism.[9] Released in early 2014, the *CLER Pathways to Excellence* is a guide addressing each of these focus areas.[9] It incorporates findings and input from the initial site visits in order to provide support for the development of these educational initiatives going forward. Much like the core competencies of the NAS, the 6 focus areas of the CLER were broken down into a series of defined pathways thought to be essential to creating an optimal clinical learning environment (**Box 2**). These pathways are further defined by a series of key properties that can be assessed at the resident/fellow, faculty, and system-wide level. In addition to providing specific learning expectations, these pathways will help guide future CLER site visits.

Early observations of CLER site visits have helped identify some strengths and weaknesses in trainee engagement in QI and safety. Generally speaking, the health care workforce, including administration and staff, seem to be very motivated to enhance the clinical learning environment and maintain a high level of commitment to GME.[10,11] Residents and fellows are taking an active role in QI and patient safety projects; but their level of involvement is highly variable and compartmentalized, often not in collaboration with system-wide efforts.[10,11] For example, at one site visit it was recognized that the residents and nurses were using the patient safety reporting system as a punitive measure as opposed to a means to improvement.[12] An area in which

---

Box 2
CLER pathways to excellence: patient safety and health care quality–related pathways

Focus Area	Pathway
Patient safety	Reporting of adverse events, close calls
	Education on patient safety
	Culture of safety
	Resident/fellow experience in patient safety investigations and follow-up
	Clinical site monitoring of resident/fellow engagement in patient safety
	Clinical site monitoring of faculty member engagement in patient safety
	Resident/fellow education and experience in disclosure of events
Health care quality	Education on QI
	Resident/fellow engagement in QI activities
	Residents/fellows receive data on quality metrics
	Residents/fellow engagement in planning for QI
	Resident/fellow and faculty member education on reducing health care disparities
	Resident/fellow engagement in clinical site initiatives to address health care disparities

Adapted from Accreditation Council for Graduate Medical Education. CLER Pathways to Clinical Excellence. 2014. Available at: http://www.acqme.org/acqmeweb/Portals/0/PDFs/CLER/_CLER_Brochure.pdf. Accessed August 6, 2015.

---

it was noted that there is a particular lack of trainee engagement is in patient safety initiatives.[10,11] Also noted was a lack of involvement in the process of safety event analysis and action plan development, with many faculty members and chief residents having never been part of a root cause/systems-based analysis.[10–12] With the data gathered from site visits, the CLER program is working toward creating targeted programs and learning materials to support continued improvement of the clinical learning environment.[10]

CURRICULAR APPROACHES TO TEACHING QUALITY IMPROVEMENT AND PATIENT SAFETY

Academic institutions are now being held accountable for integrating dedicated QI and patient safety curricula into the learning experience. The ACGME has provided the framework and essential competencies for quality and safety within the NAS to guide and support educators. It is the responsibility of educators to develop and implement programs to teach these competencies. There has been a recent push to gain new insight and knowledge regarding best practices for incorporating QI and patient safety into the educational experience of residents and fellows.

The question of how to best deliver QI and patient safety training to trainees has been addressed in 2 relatively recent systematic reviews. Both used a review model consistent with the Best Evidence Medical Education review protocol[13] to extract data and assess quality for each identified study. This protocol allows for classification of learning outcomes by Kirkpatrick's model,[13] which is a model used within many professions as a measure of effectiveness of a training program. Both reviews targeted English-language studies with residents or medical students as subjects and did not exclude any specialties.

The first review was by Wong and colleagues[14] and identified 41 studies published between January 2000 and January 2009, 27 of which included resident trainees. Although specifics varied greatly among the published studies, they were each categorized into 3 main types: teaching alone/didactic sessions, mixed didactic and experiential learning, and Web-based curricula.[14,15] The core educational content was most commonly composed of root cause analysis, systems thinking, general patient safety concepts, and error reporting.[14] Of the studies that targeted residents, the educational content was incorporated into core rotations approximately half of the time, with the other half being during independent rotations or stand-alone sessions.[14] Although only 2 of the studies demonstrated a measured benefit to patients, most of the resident-focused studies were able to report improvement in clinical processes, such as increased screening tests for patients with diabetes and increased immunizations in a pediatric clinic.[14] Although all curricular designs were effective in relaying knowledge and information regarding safety and QI concepts, the curricula that demonstrated an impact on clinical processes and patient care all had an experiential component.[14,15]

The second systematic review by Kirkman and colleagues[16] was a review of studies published between January 2009 and May 2014, 15 of which involved residents. The number of publications identified over this time period, shorter than the prior review, suggests an increasing interest in the development and subsequent evaluation of QI and patient safety curricula for trainees. In addition to root cause/systems-based analysis and general patient safety concepts, this review found a trend toward inclusion of communication and teamwork, QI, and human factors in the core curricular content.[16] The investigators thought this might relate to the increasing recognition of communication and teamwork as a critical component of achieving patient safety.[16] Most of the studies did use experiential learning and recognized the importance of striking a balance between didactic and experiential teaching.[16]

Both reviews included discussion regarding barriers and facilitators to success and sustainability of QI and patient safety curricula for trainees. The most common barriers identified across the literature included lack of faculty interest and expertise, competing time commitments, and a lack of support.[14–16] They highlighted the need for greater investment in faculty development for purposes of achieving a sufficient number of instructors as well as ensuring good physician role models during daily clinical teaching. It was suggested that patient safety and QI education be taught at a time free from competing clinical commitments, as many residents did not complete projects simply because of not having enough time. Another option to overcoming time limitations is to have the trainees participate in hospital-initiated projects as opposed to their own de novo project. This option was demonstrated in a study out of Seattle Children's Hospital that showed an increased rate of resident participation in QI activities with this approach.[17] The reviews also identified that the success of implementing these curricula depend on having adequate personnel and financial and technological resources. Without this support, many QI projects become frustrating and infeasible for trainees, lessening the value of the learning experience.

What is the optimal format for incorporating QI and patient safety into the educational curriculum? Ultimately, it will be unique to each program and will depend on the goals of teaching and the support of the clinical training environment. Evidence suggests that teaching the basic principles of patient safety and QI methodology can be accomplished through didactic sessions, such as lectures, or Web-based modules. Incorporating QI projects into the curriculum can be challenging logistically but has been shown to further engage learners and help facilitate the development of application skills.

EXPERIENCES IN TEACHING QUALITY IMPROVEMENT AND SAFETY TO PEDIATRIC TRAINEES

Some pediatric training programs have published their experiences in educating and involving trainees in QI and patient safety efforts.

Cincinnati Children's Hospital Medical Center has been one of the pioneers in involving residents and fellows in improvement and safety initiatives. Philibert and colleagues[18] published their institutional experiences with the development and implementation of a sustainable QI and patient safety curriculum for pediatric residents. In this article, they discuss the various curricular approaches they have used as well as offer practical guidance for other programs wishing to enhance their QI curriculum. All of their approaches combine teaching of the basic principles of improvement science with personal project development. They describe the results of their continued efforts to teach and involve their residents in QI initiatives, which include a month-long rotation focusing on QI as well as incorporation of improvement science into routine day-to-day hospital activities. The required general pediatric inpatient rotation allows for QI education and resident-driven improvement of patient care. The curriculum consists of improvement science methodology and tools taught in a conference setting by faculty with QI expertise.[18] Residents also become involved in short projects that are often completed in teams and allow for practical application of their newly learned skills. In order to integrate QI learning into daily training, the residents are encouraged to participate in activities, such as morning safety huddles and reviews of medical response team activations. From their experiences, the investigators present 5 concepts for programs to consider when they are looking to further enhance the QI learning during residency (**Box 3**).

Box 3
Five concepts to enhance resident learning and application of QI skills

Concepts	Effective Interventions

Enhancing QI education models and modules to ensure an appropriate grounding in QI principles
 	
Faculty development for teaching and applying QI in the clinical setting
	Teaching materials through Institute for Healthcare Improvement's Open School (www.ihi.org)
	• Set of nested training courses:
	  ○ Online modules
	  ○ Courses designed to teach advanced QI concepts and methods, leadership, and research skills
	  ○ Postdoctoral training program for fellows and junior faculty
	
	• Have core group receive training with goal of disseminating to others

Ensuring that all residents receive QI education	• Interactive workshops held after hours • Required rotation dedicated to QI concept and experiential learning
Overcoming time and opportunity constraints to allow residents to apply newly developed QI skills by incorporating them in daily residents routines	• Protected time from other clinical duties • Projects that are feasible to complete in short time period • Projects addressing problems that affect patients' or trainees' daily lives
Assessing the effect of residents' QI exposure on competence and project outcomes	Systems QI training and assessment tool

Adapted from Philibert I, Gonzalez Del Rey JA, Lannon C, et al. Quality improvement skills for pediatric residents: from lecture to implementation and sustainability. Acad Pediatr 2014;14(1):40–6.

The pediatric residency program at The University of California, Davis published the strategies and outcomes of their QI curriculum.[19] They designed a primarily experiential program aimed at enhancing residents' comfort with applying QI through team-based projects. The curriculum evolved over a 3-year period of time in response to resident feedback, implemented through plan-do-study-act (PDSA) cycles. The third year of the program, determined to be optimal for resident education in QI at their institution based on feedback, consisted of small teams of first-year residents mentored by senior residents and faculty members. Team projects were chosen from a list that focused on areas aligned with organizational priorities. Education on QI science was completed through the Institute for Healthcare Improvement Open School Web site. Results of their statistical analysis showed significant improvement in comfort level with QI concepts in first-year residents, although engaging the senior residents in additional training did not confer any additional measurable benefit in their comfort level. They discussed another benefit to the design of their curriculum, which was the pairing of faculty mentors with no experience in QI with those with expertise in the area, which helped promote faculty development.

The use of PDSA cycles to bring about continuous educational improvement in QI curriculums is a method that has been used by other programs. For example, residents and fellows rotating through the medical intensive care unit at Henry Ford Hospital in Detroit, Michigan were provided with education on PDSA methodology and then challenged to apply these principles to PDSA activities focused on improving clinical outcomes, such as iatrogenic pneumothorax rates and sepsis-specific mortality.[20] This approach allowed them to integrate, measure, and improve both educational and clinical outcomes in an ongoing process. By linking competency-based learning to clinical outcomes, trainees were able to gain knowledge and experience of QI processes while improving patient care.

The pediatric neurology residency program out of Boston Children's Hospital developed a QI and patient safety curriculum to address the QI and patient safety-related ACGME core competencies.[21] Their devised curriculum consisted of faculty-led lectures and mentored QI projects that took place over a 9-month period. The projects were completed in teams and culminated in a short presentation to faculty, whom evaluated their projects using a standardized form. Residents were surveyed before and after the 9-month intervention period and showed improved confidence in their QI project development skills, and almost twice as many residents thought they were prepared to make improvements in their practice after completing the curriculum. They identified the important characteristics of the program to be the presence of faculty mentors, incorporation of teaching into a core lecture series, provision of time to complete projects, department support, and a structured evaluation process. All of this was done with the understanding that a strong infrastructure involving processes and well-trained faculty was essential to the successful training of residents and fellows.

When developing a quality and safety curriculum for their neonatology fellows, the neonatology department at Boston Children's Hospital created a program with key elements and themes that relied on the unique features of fellowship training.[22] Recognizing that fellows' primary scholarly focus should be their research, they created a program that integrated quality and safety learning and projects within the existing clinical experiences. If possible, they tied concepts of quality and safety into the fellows' scholarly research. The curriculum encompassed the entire 3 years of fellowship, during which time the fellows were expected to complete a series of Web-based modules, lecture-based workshops, and a QI project. This longitudinal experience was supported by the fellowship structure, which typically offers a more continuous experience compared with the typical residency organization of month-long block rotations. Additionally, many fellowship programs start out with heavy clinical responsibilities and then shift the focus to research and academics near the end of training. This framework is conducive to the natural progression of a QI project, such as the PDSA cycle. For these reasons and others, the investigators concluded that fellowship training is particularly well suited for trainee engagement in system-wide QI initiatives.

In the authors' pediatric emergency department (PED), they established an Interdivisional Emergency Department Peer Review Committee whose responsibilities have included, among others, monthly reviews of (a) return visits to the PED within 72 hours with appropriate review of literature and dissemination of relevant information regarding current guidelines and updates among practitioners, (b) medication errors (in ordering and dispensing), (c) intensive care unit transfers of patients within 12 hours of admission to the general floor from the PED, (d) mortality and morbidity review, (e) radiology call backs and misses, and lastly, development of protocols for specific conditions with the aim of enhancing and promoting patient safety. This interdisciplinary committee includes PED faculty, nursing leadership, fellows in training, and research coordinators. As part of their training, fellows are assigned along with a supervising faculty member to one or more of the activities (first year of training, return visits and peer review; second year, pharmacy medication errors, protocol development, and radiology call backs; and third year, intensive care unit transfers and mortality and morbidity cases). After a review of both the cases and literature, fellows present and discuss them at these meetings. Any protocol development is done with an assigned faculty member, presented at the meeting, and then instituted at a divisional or departmental level. Active role in this mandated activity has resulted in multiple QI projects spearheaded by fellows, published research projects, faculty development processes, and multicenter trials and has been of tremendous educational value to the fellows. Further feedback about the activity and the curriculum itself from the fellows in training for the past 8 years since implementation has been extremely positive.

STATE OF QUALITY IMPROVEMENT AND PATIENT SAFETY EDUCATION IN PEDIATRIC GRADUATE MEDICAL EDUCATION

It has now been more than a decade since medical education accreditation bodies started emphasizing the importance of educating our future physicians on issues related to QI, patient safety, and systems-level thinking. Despite an increased recognition of the need to teach QI and patient safety to trainees, the implementation has been slow, likely hindered by barriers to success and a general lack of understanding of how to best teach this emerging focus within medicine. In order to continue to move forward, we must assess the current roles of QI and patient safety within pediatric GME. To accomplish this, surveys completed by both pediatric program directors and pediatric residents have been collected and analyzed.

To gain insight into how programs have been incorporating QI and patient safety into the educational framework, a survey was distributed to all pediatric program directors at the end of 2011.[23] Of the 104 programs that responded, 85% had a QI curriculum. Of those with programs, a majority included an experiential component, but fewer than half provided residents with project support. Program content varied widely in the specific process methodologies and tools that they taught as part of the curriculum. The methods used to evaluate the effectiveness of the QI programs were very inconsistent, with some programs having no method. Although most program directors thought resident participation in hospital-based initiatives was important, less than a quarter reported their residents to be involved in them. Only a minority of residency program directors described being satisfied with their current curriculum.

Fellowship training provides a unique opportunity for subspecialty-focused, longitudinal QI and patient safety education for trainees. Yet evidence suggests that, much like pediatric residency program directors, fellowship directors are also struggling to integrate it into their curriculum. Pediatric emergency medicine is a particularly vulnerable area for threats to patient safety. Large volumes and increasing pressure to see patients rapidly coupled with trainees of all levels rotating from different programs in an environment that includes multiple handoffs, weight-based dose calculations and various shift timings makes the emergency department a perfect recipe for potential disasters in patient safety. In a survey of pediatric emergency medicine program directors, Wolf and colleagues[24] noted that only 24.6% of programs reported having a formal safety curriculum. Further, compared with pediatric fellowship programs, general emergency departments reported a higher number of safety programs for residents. Program directors reported that fellows spend a median of 6 hours during their fellowship on the curriculum. Didactic sessions and case-based learning were the most commonly used formats and methodology. This survey highlights the void in this area and an urgent need for improved training of pediatric emergency fellows in safety and quality curriculum.

Third-year categorical pediatric residents across the United States were surveyed in spring 2013 regarding their experiences and perceptions of their QI curriculum.[25] Many residents reported that their residency's QI program was well organized, prepared them to perform QI projects, and met their learning needs. Most residents did participate in projects, but more than 30% did not receive any feedback on their work. Most residents were generally satisfied with their QI training. Perhaps the most encouraging result was that 84% of respondents endorsed an intention to use QI methods and skills after residency.

These surveys, although admittedly performed more than 1 year apart, show a large discordance between program directors' and residents' perceptions. This discordance could be explained by a limitation of the resident survey, which was a voluntary survey only distributed to residents whose program directors agreed to participate. This point raises the possibility of a skewed sample, with those program directors with a less developed curriculum or less interest in QI being less likely to agree to participation. However, study design limitations aside, it is possible that QI and patient safety education had a punctuated period of growth and development in the time between surveys. The fact that pediatrics was introduced and started the transition to the NAS during that period of time supports this theory. However, one must also consider that many residents are introduced to QI methodology as novices and could be overestimating their proficiency and readiness. One conclusion that could be drawn from both surveys is that there is a general lack of assessment and feedback regarding resident learning and participation in QI. This deficiency is likely a result of a lack of instruments available to measure QI outcomes and objectively assess gains in residents' QI skills, knowledge, and behavior. Currently, one such assessment tool that has been tested on pediatric residents is the Quality Improvement Knowledge Application Tool, which was able to detect a statistically significant improvement in residents' QI knowledge acquisition after curricular instruction.[26]

A group from the University of Massachusetts Medical School has studied pediatric resident training about medical errors and their prevention.[27,28] They conducted a national survey of pediatric chief residents regarding the amount and type of training that pediatric residents have about medical errors. In the initial survey in 2002, they found pediatric resident training on medical errors to be inconsistent and variable, with only 50% reporting a formalized curriculum.[27] By the 2010 survey, 94% had a formalized curriculum to discuss medical errors.[28] Although in 2002 many of the chief residents identified one-on-one talks or discussions as the primary mode of education, in 2010 they described more formalized teaching settings, including morbidity and mortality conferences, morning reports, lectures, and intern orientations. As they discuss in their report on the 2010 survey, this positive change was somewhat to be expected given the timely transition over to the NAS, which focuses on the teaching of error identification and implementation of systems-based solutions through its SBP core competency. One notable discrepancy discussed by the investigators was regarding the discussion of medical errors occurring in the outpatient versus inpatient setting. Although 72% of chief residents in 2010 reported that they discuss medical errors in the inpatient setting often, 92% reported they never or rarely discussed medical errors in the outpatient setting. Given the large proportion of pediatric residents that go on to have careers in a private practice or clinic setting, it is crucial that patient safety discussions and QI improvement opportunities for trainees extend beyond the hospital setting.

SUMMARY

Physicians in training play an integral role in QI and patient safety outcomes. Not only are they often at the forefront of patient care but they also interact with all members of a health care team, making their active participation and involvement in organizational improvement initiatives crucial to their success. As a fundamental part of the health care milieu, it is really not a question of *if* residents and fellows should be involved in the betterment of a health care system, but rather *how* to best prepare them for success in this role.

Although some academic institutions recognized the need to engage residents and fellows in QI early on, others are just now beginning to develop a formal educational curriculum. The NAS and CLER pathways developed by the ACGME provide a framework for what should be taught but do not impose strict guidelines to allow for innovation and flexibility within the heterogeneous training environments, which has resulted in great variability in curricular content and organization. As programs continue to develop, revise, and refine, it is imperative that they rigorously evaluate their effectiveness.

Much remains to be discovered about optimizing trainee engagement in QI and patient safety. Many aspects of the topic still remain areas ripe for research: optimal curricular content and a validated tool for measuring curricular impact, to name a few. The ultimate question will be whether GME's push toward an enhanced QI and patient safety education for trainees translates into changed behaviors and increased involvement later on in a physician's career. At this point, we can only hope that by sowing the seeds of safe and quality care early on, our next generation of physicians will continue to cultivate positive change.

REFERENCES

1. Leape LL, Berwick DM. Five years after to err is human: what have we learned? JAMA 2005;293(19):2384–90.
2. Macy J Jr. Foundation. Ensuring an effective physician workforce for the United States: recommendations for reforming graduate medical education to meet the needs of the public: conference summary. 2011. Available at: http://macyfoundation.org/docs/macy_pubs/JMF_GME_Conference2_Monograph(2).pdf. Accessed August 8, 2015.

3. Nasca TJ, Philibert I, Brigham T, et al. The next GME accreditation system–rationale and benefits. N Engl J Med 2012;366(11):1051–6.

4. Accreditation Council for Graduate Medical Education. ACGME common program requirements. Chicago: Accreditation Council for Graduate Medical Education; 2013.

5. Accreditation Council for Graduate Medical Education. Next Accreditation System (NAS). 2013. Available at: https://www.acgme.org/acgmeweb/tabid/143/ProgramandInstitutionalAccreditation/MedicalSpecialties/Pediatrics.aspx. Accessed August 3, 2015.

6. Accreditation Council for Graduate Medical Education. Pediatric Milestones Project. 2013. Available at: https://www.acgme.org/acgmeweb/Portals/0/PDFs/Milestones/320_PedsMilestonesProject.pdf. Accessed August 3, 2015.

7. American Academy of Pediatrics. The medical home. Pediatrics 2002;110:184–6.

8. Weiss KB, Wagner R, Nasca TJ. Development, testing, and implementation of the ACGME Clinical Learning Environment Review (CLER) program. J Grad Med Educ 2012;4(3):396–8.

9. Accreditation Council for Graduate Medical Education. CLER pathways to clinical excellence. 2014. Available at: https://www.acgme.org/acgmeweb/Portals/0/PDFs/CLER/CLER_Brochure.pdf. Accessed August 6, 2015.

10. Weiss KB, Wagner R, Bagian JP, et al. Advances in the ACGME Clinical Learning Environment Review (CLER) program. J Grad Med Educ 2013;5(4):718–21.

11. Accreditation Council for Graduate Medical Education. CLER pathways to clinical excellence. 2014. Available at: http://www.acgme.org/acgmeweb/Portals/0/PDFs/CLER/CLERProgramUpdateWebinar10-11-13.pdf. Accessed August 6, 2015.

12. Weiss KB, Bagian JP, Nasca TJ. The clinical learning environment: the foundation of graduate medical education. JAMA 2013;309(16):1687–8.

13. Hammick M, Dornan T, Steinert Y. Conducting a best evidence systematic review. Part 1: from idea to data coding. BEME guide No. 13. Med Teach 2010; 32:3–15.

14. Wong BM, Etchells EE, Kuper A, et al. Teaching quality improvement and patient safety to trainees: a systematic review. Acad Med 2010;85(9):1425–39.

15. Wong BM, Levinson W, Shojania KG. Quality improvement in medical education: current state and future directions. Med Educ 2012;46(1):107–19.

16. Kirkman MA, Sevdalis N, Arora S, et al. The outcomes of recent patient safety education interventions for trainee physicians and medical students: a systematic review. BMJ Open 2015;5(5):1–17.

17. Lipstein EA, Kronman MP, Richmond C, et al. Addressing core competencies through hospital quality improvement activities: attitudes and engagement. J Grad Med Educ 2011;3(3):315–9.

18. Philibert I, Gonzalez Del Rey JA, Lannon C, et al. Quality improvement skills for pediatric residents: from lecture to implementation and sustainability. Acad Pediatr 2014;14(1):40–6.

19. Shaikh U, Natale JE, Nettiksimmons J, et al. Improving pediatric health care delivery by engaging residents in team-based quality improvement projects. Am J Med Qual 2013;28(2):120–6.

20. Buckley JD, Joyce B, Garcia AJ, et al. Linking residency training effectiveness to clinical outcomes: a quality improvement approach. Jt Comm J Qual Patient Saf 2010;36(5):203–8.

21. Maski KP, Loddenkemper T, An S, et al. Development and implementation of a quality improvement curriculum for child neurology residents: lessons learned. Pediatr Neurol 2014;50(5):452–7.

22. Gupta M, Ringer S, Tess A, et al. Developing a quality and safety curriculum for fellows: lessons learned from a neonatology fellowship program. Acad Pediatr 2014;14(1):47–53.

23. Mann KJ, Craig MS, Moses JM. Quality improvement educational practices in pediatric residency programs: survey of pediatric program directors. Acad Pediatr 2014;14(1):23–8.

24. Wolff M, Macias CG, Garcia E, et al. Patient safety training in pediatric emergency medicine: a national survey of program directors. Acad Emerg Med 2014;21(7): 835–8.

25. Craig MS, Garfunkel LC, Baldwin CD, et al. Pediatric resident education in quality improvement (QI): a national survey. Acad Pediatr 2014;14(1):54–61.

26. Glissmeyer EW, Ziniel SI, Moses J. Use of the quality improvement (QI) knowledge application tool in assessing pediatric resident QI education. J Grad Med Educ 2014;6(2):284–91.

27. Walsh KE, Miller MR, Vinci RJ, et al. Pediatric resident education about medical errors. Ambul Pediatr 2004;4(6):514–7.

28. Bradley CK, Fischer MA, Walsh KE. Trends in medical error education: are we failing our residents? Acad Pediatr 2013;13(1):59–64.

Clinical Pathways
Driving High-Reliability and High-Value Care

Andrew R. Buchert, MD[a],*, Gabriella A. Butler, MSN, RN[b]

KEYWORDS

- Pathways • Clinical pathways • Guidelines • High reliability • Triple aim
- Outcomes measurement

KEY POINTS

- Health care in the United States is largely delivered in systems of care that are complex, inefficient, error prone, and costly. There currently exists a high degree of variability in the delivery of care between providers and settings of care. Other industries outside of health care have been successful at reducing inefficiencies and eliminating waste through the standardization of processes. Clinical pathways allow for an opportunity to reduce variability in the delivery of health care.
- Clinical pathways can have positive impact on the quality of care delivered to individual patients, on the health of populations of patients with particular diseases or conditions, on the workflow of frontline providers, and on processes within the health care organization. Additionally, clinical pathways can drive positive economic results and can have impact on advancing the strategic mission of the health care organization.
- Clinical pathways will be most successful if they are interdisciplinary and multidisciplinary, if they are evidence-based as well as consensus-based for the local health care environment, if there is the ability to engage in ongoing and real-time measurement with a commitment to making results actionable, and if the pathways are aligned with the strategy of the organization.
- The potential barriers to the successful implementation of clinical pathways can often be negated by a commitment to both the development and the sustainability of the pathway by all levels of the organization.

Disclosures: None.
[a] Clinical Resource Management & Education Outreach, Children's Hospital of Pittsburgh of UPMC, Donald D Wolff Center for Quality, Safety, and Innovation, University of Pittsburgh School of Medicine, 4401 Penn Avenue, Pittsburgh, PA 15224, USA; [b] Clinical Resource Management, Solutions for Patient Safety, Clinical Quality Analytics, Children's Hospital of Pittsburgh of UPMC, 4401 Penn Avenue, Pittsburgh, PA 15224, USA
* Corresponding author.
E-mail address: Andrew.Buchert@chp.edu

Pediatr Clin N Am 63 (2016) 317–328
http://dx.doi.org/10.1016/j.pcl.2015.12.005
0031-3955/16/$ – see front matter
pediatric.theclinics.com

INTRODUCTION

Health care providers and consumers in the United States exist in a system that is fraught with errors, inconsistencies, and inefficiencies. The Institute of Medicine has estimated that nearly 100,000 people die every year because of medical errors.[1] It is also known that the US health care system remains one of the most costly in the world.[2] There is much to be learned from those industries outside of health care that have come to be known as high-reliability organizations. Of the many qualities that set apart these industries as leaders and innovators in error reduction and process improvement, one of the overriding themes embraced by these industries is a reduction of variability.[3] Lean methodology derived from the Toyota Production System, as well as six sigma, were developed by and employed in the manufacturing industry for process improvement. Both of these methodologies are now being applied in many service industries as well as within health care.

The complexity of the health care industry allows for many opportunities to reduce variability through the standardization of numerous processes. There are many nonclinical processes within health care that are analogous to the manufacturing industry to which these types of methodologies can readily be applied (eg, central sterilization and laboratory specimen receiving and processing). The application of such methodologies to clinical care, however, may seem less intuitive because of the dynamic presentation of diseases and patients' response to medical treatment. Clinical care has historically been seen as highly individualized, with clinical judgment and medical decision making solely owned by each health care provider and tailored specifically to each individual patient.[4]

Certainly, the human factor is unique to the practice of medicine, and unlike cars on a production line, an industry that specializes in taking care of people will inherently encompass situations in which variability cannot be negated. The key, however, is to focus on the reduction of inappropriate or unnecessary variation, which often occurs when care is not evidence-based or clinical decisions are not based on specific clinical factors. Standardization begins by a focus on evidence-based care in the context of the individual patient's clinical picture.[5]

As evidence-based medicine has become paramount to medical decision making and clinical judgment, there is strong support for the standardization of the delivery of clinical care.[6] The development of clinical pathways is an example of a strategy to reduce variability.

In addition to the reduction of variability, clinical pathways have direct impact on the care of individual patients, including improved quality of care and improved safety.[7] Clinical pathways can also impact the population of patients with a specific disease or condition, including streamlining ambulatory care and potentially reducing emergency department and urgent care center visits, reducing hospital admissions, and reducing readmissions by ensuring that patients are discharged with the right resources and that they have appropriate and timely postdischarge follow-up. Combined, adherence to the elements of a pathway lead to an overall reduction in the cost of health care.[8] Thus, clinical pathways fulfill each component of The Triple Aim, as defined by the Institute for Healthcare Improvement.[9]

This article will define clinical pathways and further describe the elements and tools that are necessary to successfully implement and sustain clinical pathways.

Making a Case for Pathways: a Rapidly Changing Environment and its Effect on the Evolution of Health Care

The very challenges that necessitate a new approach to the delivery of care in the United States also serve as the barriers. The spending on health care is increasing, but the pool of money to fund that spending is decreasing. Health care spending is on the rise. It is estimated that 86% of health care expenditures is used for the treatment of chronic conditions, which currently account for almost half of the population.[10] As modern medicine advances, people are living longer with chronic conditions, many of which were formerly untreatable, especially within pediatrics. Furthermore, chronic diseases will be the leading cause of death for 59% of mortalities in developing countries by the year 2030.[11] The increase in complexity of patients, as well as the aging population, forces one to realize that the current state is not sustainable.

The demand for fiscal stewardship among health organizations by federal and private payers, as well as the general public, has led to a tenuous economic climate for health care providers. Additionally, there is growing public demand for complete transparency for quality of care, outcomes, patient safety, and cost.[12] In this environment, hospitals struggle to find the balance between providing high-value care, and reducing resource utilization (**Fig. 1**).

Clinical Pathways Defined—Beyond the Algorithm

Clinical pathways are intended to reduce variability, and thus it is somewhat ironic that there is considerable variation in how clinical pathways have been defined. Often used interchangeably with clinical guidelines, protocols, care pathways, care maps, and critical pathways, it is not surprising that the definition of what constitutes clinical pathways varies among institutions.[13]

In a recent Cochrane review of the impact of clinical pathways in hospitals, researchers recognized the considerable variability in the definition of clinical

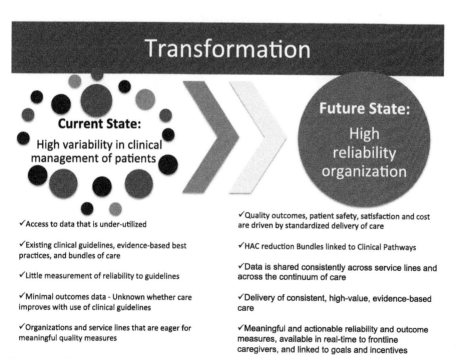

Fig. 1. Transformation to a high reliable organization via clinical pathways.

pathways.[14] They identified 5 criteria that were common to clinical pathways among the publications describing their use:

1. The intervention was a structured multidisciplinary plan of care
2. The intervention was used to channel the translation of guidelines or evidence into local structures.
3. The intervention detailed the steps in a course of treatment or care in a plan, pathway, algorithm, guideline, protocol or other inventory of actions.
4. The intervention had timeframes or criteria-based progression (that is, steps were taken if designated criteria were met).
5. The intervention aimed to standardize care for a specific clinical problem, procedure, or episode of health care in a specific population.

The authors have used the criteria as derived from the Cochran review, as a foundation to develop our proposal for the elements of a successful pathway (**Fig. 2**).

INTERDISCIPLINARY AND MULTIDISCIPLINARY

A successful pathway should be both interdisciplinary as well as multidisciplinary. The pathway should clearly delineate the elements of care specific to each discipline or role, such that there is a structured plan of care to be enacted by each member of the health care team. At the same time, the pathway will promote collaboration between the disciplines by engaging each member and ensuring each member's role as an integral member of the team. Thus, clinical pathways result in a transformation

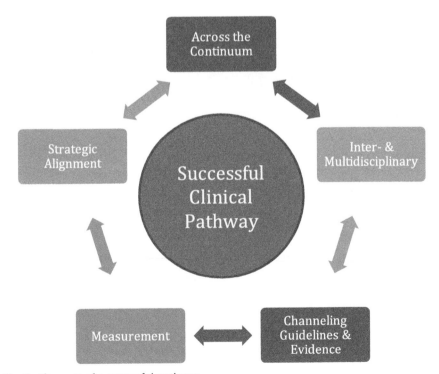

Fig. 2. Elements of a successful pathway.

from separate and parallel components of care to care that is seamlessly integrated within and between disciplines.

ACROSS THE CONTINUUM OF CARE

Not only is it important for this integration of care to occur among disciplines within one particular setting of care, it is equally as important for care to be aligned between different settings of care across the entire continuum. The treatment of diseases and medical conditions is rarely limited to 1 episode of care in 1 particular setting, but rather there is a spectrum of care that is delivered at varying levels based on the severity of the disease, the evolution and progression of the illness, and the setting of care. Care in each of these settings should be evidence-based, and there should be consistency between these varying settings and levels of care such that all providers are following the same best practice for their particular level and setting of care. This is often where true or perceived differences in the management of a particular disease or condition occur, and these differences can not only be confusing to patients, families, and providers, but can also be contradicting, dissatisfying, and frustrating.[15] These differences in care may include unnecessary testing or treatments or contradictory explanations or rationales of care, and this can result in dissatisfaction as well as loss of confidence in providers. Clinical pathways provide a vehicle to standardize the care for particular diseases or conditions such that all providers are on the same page and are providing care at their level or setting that represents a piece of the management of that particular disease or condition. As the patient moves between settings and levels of care, this consistency is continued.

In today's health care environment, care is increasingly fragmented, and providers are often disconnected between settings of care.[16] Patients and families as care consumers expect the delivery of care to function in tandem, too, and with the different pieces of care connected. The culture of today's technology-rich society is one of complete transparency and immediacy of the availability of information.[17] Health care consumers are keen to recognize when aspects of care differ between providers and care settings. This inconsistent and unpredictable care can be a significant dissatisfier. Pathways that are designed across the continuum of care can ensure that no matter where a patient's care is taking place, the delivery of that care will be based on that patient's condition and not based on the provider's preference.

As a final note, pathways should also include a map for the transition of care at each juncture, thus ensuring the seamless transfer of patient information between providers and levels of care.

CHANNELING GUIDELINES AND EVIDENCE

The process of developing and maintaining each clinical pathway provides an opportunity to examine and re-examine the literature for evidence-based best practices, and to establish local consensus on best practices and local standards. The clinical pathway should be based on evidence, as well as the specifics of the local environment and the realities of local practice.

MEASUREMENT BEYOND THE OUTCOMES

By reducing variability in clinical care, pathways exemplify the principles of high reliability, as outlined by Weick and Sutcliffe in their book, *Managing the Unexpected*.[18] Additionally, the pathways process itself is an outstanding model of incorporating the principles of high reliability.[19] The development of clinical pathways represents 1 way that organizations exhibit a preoccupation with failure. The process of developing a pathway involves complex planning for instances in which the pathway may not apply, or where patients who should be on the pathway could be missed. As pathways are by and for the frontline staff and providers, and are also built and tested by the frontlines, they represent an opportunity for organizations to employ sensitivity to operations. Pathways must account for numerous levels of complexity, as well as multiple scenarios that may occur throughout a patient's care, and so pathway development must involve a reluctance to simplify interpretations. Pathways are built to be sustainable and provide consistency, predictability, and efficiency to care, thus they are integral to an organization's commitment to resilience. Finally, pathways are built, sustained, and enacted by the frontline staff, and thus they are clearly an example of deference to expertise.

In order to ensure that clinical pathways are providing momentum to an organization's drive to high reliability, the authors suggest that clinical pathways must be measured for reliability, including caregivers' ability to adhere to essential steps in the plan of care, in addition to continuous monitoring of clinical and economic outcomes. The ability to measure and provide feedback to providers regarding adherence and outcomes is essential.

STRATEGIC ALIGNMENT

Finally, the authors suggest that clinical pathways represent an opportunity to advance the strategic mission and goals of the organization. This point will be discussed in detail further in this article.

GETTING TO THE FUTURE STATE: CLINICAL PATHWAYS MAPPING THE WAY TO HIGH-VALUE CARE

The goal of pathways is to provide consistent, safe, efficient, effective, and timely care that will yield positive patient outcomes while reducing the inappropriate use of unnecessary resources. In the report, *Crossing the Quality Chasm*, the Institute of Medicine advocates health care organizations to embrace 6 aims for improvement of patient care. The adoption of clinical pathways directly supports their proposal.[20]

PATIENT SAFETY, EFFECTIVENESS, AND EQUITABILITY

By streamlining patient care and following evidence-based pathways, patients are not otherwise exposed to medications, treatments, and tests that are unnecessary and may in fact place them at additional risk for harm. The benefit-to-risk ratio is shifted by ensuring that patients are only exposed to the care that is, necessary, and thus not exposed to aspects of care that will not improve their condition. Furthermore, clinical decisions that determine patient care should be based on relevant and high quality findings.[21] Patients, regardless of individual demographics, beliefs, and insurance status, can also be assured that their care is consistent with other patients with the same health conditions.

EFFICIENT AND TIMELY

The use of clinical pathways optimizes resource utilization, thereby reducing waste caused by unnecessary testing, procedures, and supplies. Additionally, nonvalue-added activities that consume the time of patients, caregivers, and the health care organization at large are reduced.

PATIENT-CENTERED

Pathways essentially drive care that is, safe, timely, effective, efficient, and equitable. In doing so, the care provided is inherently patient-centered. In consideration for patients whose preferences or values contradict the proposed care, the pathway provides strong support that providers can confidently and expertly describe to patients and families to aid in an informed decision.

PATHWAYS AS A STRATEGIC TOOL

Although pathways provide a roadmap of care for patients with a particular disease process, the value of pathways extends beyond clinical care. In addition to developing pathways that will yield clinical benefits, the pathways that are selected must be in alignment with the strategic plan of the organization. For instance, patient populations can be selected for pathways as an opportunity to grow a particular service line. As an example, in their organization as they were developing an eating disorder program, the authors built a pathway that would draw attention to the red flags that might indicate an eating disorder, especially by primary care and subspecialty providers. The authors recognized that many presenting complaints could actually signify an eating disorder, but if this was not recognized then many of these patients would undergo extensive and expensive work-ups that were unrevealing. The authors' pathway highlighted the red flags, with the intent of identifying this particular patient population earlier, and thus growing their service line.

Pathways can also be used to funnel patients into the most appropriate care setting as early as possible, thus decreasing unnecessary utilization of resources. For example, patients with hyperbilirubinemia not requiring consideration of an exchange transfusion can likely be cared for in an acute care setting in most organizations. A clinical pathway that channels these patients into this setting can ensure that the neonatal intensive care unit (NICU) does not utilize precious intensive care resources for these patients unless they are in need of critical care. This can ensure that the NICU is available for patients who do require critical care. As an additional benefit, this also helps to build a particular unit or service line by channeling patient populations (**Table 1**).

Table 1	
Motivation for supporting clinical pathways	
Stakeholders	**Potential Benefits**
Patients and families	• Consistent plan of care among members of the care team and across different settings of care • Clear and common goals
Nurses and staff	• Predictable care plans • Enhanced workflow and efficiency • Feedback regarding performance is readily available
Physicians	• Established pathways can support clinical decision making that may be counter to the expectations of patients and families (eg, not prescribing antibiotics for a viral illness) • Continuous evaluation of reliability and outcomes provides the opportunity to measure performance
Executive leadership	• Resource utilization • Provide insight into specific processes and service lines
Organization	• Cost-effective • Provides a focused and stepwise approach toward performance excellence

HIGH-IMPACT WITH VIABLE STAKEHOLDERS
Organization

The commitment to establishing lean, six sigma, or other process improvement methodology programs has been an effective strategy for some health care organizations. The dedication of resources necessary for the examination of an entire system for opportunities can be overwhelming and unrealistic, however, due to both cost and the shear breadth of the numerous clinical and nonclinical processes within a health care organization. The development of a clinical pathway allows for a focused and intense analysis of a smaller group of processes within an organization, and has the additive advantage of integrating feedback from the point of care. Furthermore, the success of improvement efforts on a single pathway can have a downstream effect to improve other inefficiencies within the organization.

Frontline staff engagement can be enhanced by their participation in the development of and ongoing monitoring of pathways of care. In an environment where frontline staff have increasing pressures from both internal and external sources, and in which they are increasingly questioning the value of what they do, engaging them in the development of pathways helps staff to see that the care they provide each day is not only good for the patient, but that they are contributing to the greater good of the hospital. When providers know that the care that they are providing is the right care, they are more confident in the care that they are providing. Finally, when patients and families know that the care they are receiving is the agreed-upon best practice, they have greater trust of the hospital.

Executive Leadership

There are economic advantages for the reduction of waste and variability.[22]

Specifying the appropriate resources that are evidence-based for a specific disease process or diagnosis can help the organization identify approximate costs for the care of those patients. Based on the estimated costs and volume, an organization can more appropriately estimate the budgeted resources needed, as well as provide realistic perspective for the contribution of resources needed to provide optimum care for such patients and to better determine how resources within the organization should be allocated.

Physicians

To be successful, a pathway must not only have buy-in and support from leadership, but also by the frontline staff who will use the pathway at the point of care.[23] Developing pathways with the clinicians allows the opportunity to streamline work and design a workflow that is, intuitive and predictable. The right thing to do then becomes the default for care. Additionally, the use of measurement tools to track adherence to pathways as well as outcomes based on metrics specific to each pathway will provide evidence that the current pathway is effective, or provide an opportunity for further research. This data stream with meaningful outcomes measures that relate directly to clinical care can serve as a significant motivator.

Nurses and Hospital Staff

Standardized care has a positive impact on the workflow of the nursing staff and to patient flow within the health care organization.[24] In the current system, much of the care is often not dependent on the diagnosis, but rather is provider-dependent. The use of a predetermined plan allows nurses to predict the plan of care and thus organize their work and educate the family accordingly. This enhances both nursing/staff satisfaction as well as patient satisfaction, as care is less fragmented.

Patients and Families

In addition to increased patient and family satisfaction, research supports that effective communication has an impact on health outcomes, namely because it increases patients' and families' participation in care, adherence to recommendations, and self-management.[25] The development of clinical pathways allows an opportunity to build education resources that not only provide information about the disease process that will be used for discharge, but also for what they should expect from their primary care provider, indications for follow-up, signs that they are meeting their goals on the pathway, and next steps.

Organizations that can communicate the intended course of clinical care, as well as follow through with the plan, are able to provide care that is not only high in quality from a clinical perspective, but is also perceived as the highest quality by patients and families. Clinical pathways can provide this important aspect of health care delivery (**Fig. 3**).

The Pathway for Implementation Is Not Always Without its Roadblocks...

Up to this point, the focus of this article has been on the rationale for the development and implementation of clinical pathways and the significant advantages of this work to all aspects of the missions of health care organizations. The actual implementation of clinical pathways is not without it challenges, however. To be successful in the reduction of variability, pathways must drive care that is the same regardless of provider, with variability only based upon clinical factors that might necessitate deviation from the pathway. Pathways thus must be based upon an evidence-based best practice, and there must be consensus among all of the stakeholders. This may include a physician group within a specialty, physicians outside of that specialty who serve in consulting roles to the particular patients with the diagnosis or condition that the pathway addresses, physicians, and other expert staff including pharmacists, epidemiologists, and laboratory personnel who must approve certain aspects of care within the pathway such as use of a particular antibiotic, and the frontline nursing and ancillary staff who all participate in the care of the patients on the pathway. Obtaining consensus among this varied and diverse group of professionals can be daunting,

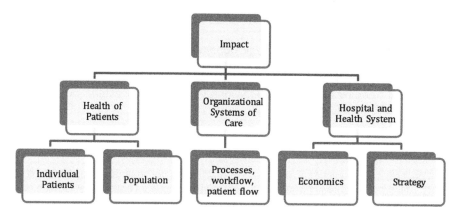

Fig. 3. Multifaceted impact of clinical pathways.

and the time course and number of meetings necessary to accomplish this may be lengthy. It may even be necessary for the pathway to ultimately include some points of diversion or variability when it becomes clear that consensus cannot be realistically obtained.

Another challenge may occur with establishing a data stream that is reliable, meaningful, timely, and actionable.[26] The authors believe that this is critical to the sustainability of a pathway, but establishing this may require significant investment of resources into information technology infrastructure and personnel, and a significant investment of time by expert clinical stakeholders such as the information technology team works to build the data stream in a way that will be timely, meaningful, and instantly actionable to frontline staff who are the owners of each particular pathway.

Maintaining the sustainability of pathways is critical, but not easy, especially after the initial excitement and energy have worn off with time. The process of developing, rolling out, and implementing a pathway involves the key stakeholders, and the associated educational campaign likely encompasses many of the frontline staff. But after the pathway has been in place for some time, there is risk that the energy and enthusiasm that surrounded the development and launching of the pathway will wane. Thus, the continuous, timely, meaningful, and actionable data stream as previously described is essential to maintain buy-in from stakeholders and to ensure the sustainability of the pathway. It is also essential that over time the evidence behind each pathway is re-evaluated to ensure that pathways are based on the most up-to-date clinical evidence. Doing this requires that the frontline staff owners of each pathway maintain commitment to continual review of the literature, and when changes are necessary that the owners re-engage all of the stakeholders to update the pathway.

SUMMARY: SUCCESSFUL CLINICAL PATHWAY IMPLEMENTATION AND SUSTAINABILITY

Having identified the barriers, the authors propose that the successful development and maintenance of clinical pathways must, at a minimum, incorporate the following 2 elements:

1. Buy-in and support at all levels of the organization, with both executive and organizational support, as well as frontline staff support and commitment to sustainability
2. A feasible ability to continually measure all aspects of the impact of the pathway, and an established feedback loop to ensure that all stakeholders are engaged in the ongoing assessment of the pathway and its impact, ideally in real time or as close to real time as is possible.

Clinical pathways represent a strategic opportunity for health care organizations to drive care that is truly high-value care, care that exemplifies the triple aim as described by the Institute for Healthcare Improvement, and care that drives high reliability throughout the organization. For these reasons, the authors suggest that clinical pathways represent the future of health care delivery.

REFERENCES

1. The Institute of Medicine. To err is human: building a safer health system. Washington, DC: National Academy Press; 1999. Available at: http://iom.nationalacademies.org/~/media/Files/Report%20Files/1999/To-Err-is-Human/To%20Err%20is%20Human%201999%20%20report%20brief.pdf.

2. World Health Organization. 2015. Health expenditure, total (% of GDP). 2015 World Bank Group. Available at: http://data.worldbank.org/indicator/SH.XPD. TOTL.ZS. Accessed December 6, 2015.

3. Neuhauser D, Provost L, Bergman B. The meaning of cariation to healthcare managers, clinical and health-services researchers, and individual patients. BMJ Qual Saf 2011;20(1):36–40.

4. May C, Rapley T, Moreira T, et al. Technogovernance: evidence, subjectivity, and the clinical encounter in primary care medicine. Soc Sci Med 2005;62:1022–30.

5. Mammen C, Mastell DG, Lemley KV. The importance of clinical pathways and protocols in pediatric nephrology. Pediatr Nephrol 2014;29:1903–14.

6. Vanhaecht K, Bollmann M, Bower K, et al. Prevalence and use of clinical pathways in 23 countries: an international survey by the European Pathway Association. Journal of Integrated Care Pathways 2006;10:28–34.

7. Wolff AM, Taylor SA, McCabe JF. Using checklists and reminders in clinical pathways to improve hospital inpatient care. Med J Aust 2004;181:428–31.

8. Share DA, Campbell DA, Birkmeyer N, et al. How a regional collaborative of hospitals and physicians in Michigan cut costs and improved the quality of care. Health Aff 2011;30:636–45.

9. Institute for Healthcare Improvement. IHI triple aim initiative: better care for individuals, better health for populations, and lower per capita costs. Cambridge (MA): IHI Initiatives Page; 2015. Available at:www.ihi.org/engage/initiatives/tripleaim/Pages/default.aspx.

10. Centers for Disease Control and Prevention. Chronic disease overview page. Available at: http://www.cdc.gov/chronicdisease. Accessed December 6, 2015.

11. Stuckler D. Population causes and consequences of leading chronic diseases: a comparative analysis of prevailing explanations. Milbank Q 2008;86(2):273–326.

12. Ball C. What is transparency? Public Integrity 2014;11(4):293–308.

13. Saint S, Hofer TP, Rose JS, et al. Use of critical pathways to improve efficiency: a cautionary tale. Am J Manag Care 2003;9:758–65.

14. Kinsman L, Rotter T, James E, et al. What is a clinical pathways? Development of a definition to inform the debate. BMC Med 2010;8:31.

15. Yeh TM, Pai FY, Huang K. Effects of clinical pathway implementation on medical quality and patient satisfaction. Total Qual Manag Bus Excel 2015;26(5/6): 582–601.

16. The Institute of Medicine. Crossing the quality chasm: a new health system for the 21st Century. Washington, DC: National Academy Press; 2001.

17. World Health Organization. Issues in health information: national and subnational health information systems. Geneva (Switzerland): World Health Organization International: Health Metrics Network; 2005. p. 1. Available at: http://www.who.int/healthmetrics/library/issue_1_05apr.doc.

18. Weick K, Sutcliffe K. Managing the unexpected: resilient performance in the age of uncertainty. 2nd edition. San Francisco (CA): John Wiley &Sons, Inc; 2007.

19. Chassin MR, Loeb JM. High-reliability health care: getting there from here. Milbank Q 2013;91(3):459–90.

20. The Institute of Medicine. Crossing the quality chasm: a new health system for the 21st century. Washington, DC: National Academy Press; 2001.

21. Brouwers M, Kho ME, Browman GP, et al. AGREE II: advancing guideline development, reporting and evaluation in healthcare. J Clin Epidemiol 2010;63: 1308–11.

22. Rotter T, Kugler J, Koch R, et al. A systematic review and meta-analysis of the effects of clinical pathways on lenth of stay, hospital costs and patient outcomes. BMC Health Serv Res 2008;8:265.

23. Silow-Carroll S, Alteras T, Meyer JA. Hospital quality improvement: strategies and lessons from U.S. hospitals. New York: Commonwealth Fund; 2007. Commonwealth Fund pub 1009. Available at: http://www.commonwealthfund. org/usr_doc/Silow-Carroll_hosp_quality_improve_strategies_lessons_1009.pdf.

24. Seehusen D. Clinical pathways: effects on practice, outcomes, and costs. Am Fam Physician 2010;82(11):1338–9.

25. Deneckere S, Euwema M, Van Herck P, et al. Care pathways lead to better teamwork: results of a systematic review. Soc Sci Med 2012;75(2):264–8.

26. Tang PC, Ralston M, Arrigotti MF, et al. Comparison of methodologies for calculating quality measures based on administrative data versus clinical data from an electronic health record system: Implications for performance measures. J Am Med Inform Assoc 2007;14(1):10–5.

Pediatric Quality and Safety: A Nursing Perspective

Gabriella A. Butler, MSN, RN[a],*, Diane S. Hupp, DNP, RN, NEA-BC[b]

KEYWORDS

- Nursing quality • Patient safety • High-reliability organization • Pediatrics
- Serious adverse events • Nursing empowerment • Quality improvement

KEY POINTS

- Although the environment of health care is continuously transforming, nurses' steadfast commitment to quality and safety must remain the priority.
- Nurses have significant influence within organizations to drive and elevate patient safety and quality, ultimately resulting in better patient outcomes.
- It is essential for nurse leaders to empower bedside nurses in the processes and initiatives on how organizations will transform their care to a safer, higher-quality delivery system while driving value/efficiency.
- To elevate commitment to patient safety and high quality, it is important for nurses to work collaboratively with other disciplines to build sustainable and uniform care processes that assist them in their delivering quality care.
- Hospital leadership must provide an environment and culture whereby nurses on the front line are actively engaged and participative in the strategy and implementation of work to improve quality and patient safety and ultimately increase transparency to drive the culture of a high-reliability organization (HRO).

INTRODUCTION

Patient safety remains a challenge among all health care providers today, including nurses. Despite increased public attention and the rise on the agendas of members of the board and C-suite executives, it is not consistently the top priority in many organizations. Adequate time has not been given to the priority of patient safety.[1,2]

As organizations are mandated to transform to value-based care, whereby volume is not the driver but rather quality and safety are higher priorities for all providers, nurses are instrumental in redefining care models to create cost efficiency while still providing safe

Disclosures: None.
[a] Clinical Resource Management, Solutions for Patient Safety, Clinical Quality Analytics, Children's Hospital of Pittsburgh of UPMC, 4401 Penn Avenue, Pittsburgh, PA 15224, USA;
[b] Patient Care Services, Children's Hospital of Pittsburgh of UPMC, 4401 Penn Avenue, Pittsburgh, PA 15224, USA
* Corresponding author.
E-mail address: Gabriella.butler@chp.edu

Pediatr Clin N Am 63 (2016) 329–339
http://dx.doi.org/10.1016/j.pcl.2015.11.005
0031-3955/16/$ – see front matter © 2016 Elsevier Inc. All rights reserved.

and high-quality care. It is critical that nurses protect patients from preventable harm. In the hospital setting, nurses are with patients 24/7/365, giving them the encouragement to speak up. Nurses are the primary advocates for their patients. For pediatric patients, a nurse may be the sole voice advocating for the child. Although the environment of health care has changed, nurses' commitment to safety and quality must take precedence.

WHAT DOES IT MEAN TO PROVIDE SAFE AND QUALITY NURSING CARE?

The nursing profession, both past and present, has maintained an intense commitment to quality and safety. More than a century ago, Florence Nightingale taught that the first requirement in a hospital is that it should do the sick no harm.[3]

The fundamental principles that Nightingale described are the same principles that nurses are educated in today. She believed hospitals should help patients, not hurt them. She set standards for hospitals to be clean and safe. These efforts are supported by the Institute of Medicine and are held in high regard by national recognition programs, including the Magnet Accreditation Program, Leapfrog Group Hospital Survey, and *U.S. News and World Report Honor Roll of Best Hospitals*. Nurses have a responsibility to their patients and families to elevate patient safety by eliminating preventable harm and delivering high quality care.

SAFETY AND QUALITY ARE AT THE CORE OF NURSING PRACTICE

The impetus for an investment in patient safety gained national attention with the Institute of Medicine's report, *To Err is Human: Building a Safer Health System* (1999).[4] The report concluded that as many as 98,000 people die each year as a result of medical errors. The subsequent report, *Crossing the Quality Chasm* (2001),[5] focused on closing the quality gap. A call for action and improvements, focusing on the six aims of health care: patient safety; effective; patient-centeredness; timeliness; care efficiency; and equity. A consistent theme in both reports was the power of nurses, both at the bedside and within the hospital leadership structure, to identify problems and develop solutions.

As the largest group of health care providers in the United States, nurses have significant influence within organizations to make improvements in each of the 6 aims **(Table 1)**. It is critical for nurses at all levels to be engaged in the processes and initiatives on how organizations transform their care to a safer, higher-quality delivery system while driving value/efficiency.

HIGH COST DOES NOT EQUATE TO HIGH QUALITY

The United States has the highest cost associated with health care as defined by the percentage of the gross domestic product (GDP) in comparison to other well-developed countries.[14] Despite the persistent increase in national spending for health care, the United States continues to underperform in comparison to other high-income countries when ranked by the Commonwealth Fund on measures of health outcomes, quality, and efficiency[15] **(Fig. 1)**.

Health care spending is projected to continue to increase at an estimated rate of 5.8% per year by 2024.[16] Furthermore, given the expansion of health insurance coverage with the implementation of the Affordable Care Act and the aging population, Centers for Medicare & Medicaid Services estimates that 47% of national health spending will be financed by the government by 2024. The etiologies of health care costs are highly complex and multifactorial.

Advances in health care have dramatically changed the landscape of chronic conditions. Diseases and conditions that were formally untreatable have become chronic

Table 1
Institute of Medicine 6 aims for improvement

Aim	Description by the Institute of Medicine	Implications for Nursing
Patient safety	Avoiding injuries to patients from the care that is intended to help them	Nurses are advocates – they maintain patient rights and support the ability of each individual to promote well-being, as defined by that individual.[6] Organizations should empower nurses to report errors and to intervene if they perceive that there is impending harm. Similarly, nurses should share this message with patients, and encourage them to take an active role in error prevention.[7]
Effective	Providing services based on scientific knowledge to all who could benefit and refraining from providing services to those not likely to benefit	The advancement of evidence-based practice in nursing supports this dimension, because organizations make clinical decisions based on the most relevant evidence and high-quality findings.[8]
Patient-centered	Providing care that is respectful of and responsive to individual patient preferences, needs, and values and ensuring that patient values guide all clinical decisions	The patient-centered care movement has challenged nurses to see health care from the patient's perspective. Models of patient-centered care include bedside handoff, interdisciplinary patient/family-centered rounds, and hourly rounding. Patient-centered care has been shown to have a positive impact on patients' optimism, sense of well-being, and trust.[9]
Timely	Reducing waits and sometimes harmful delays for both those who receive and those who give care	A systematic review of the impact of nurse staffing on cost and length of stay encourages hospitals to provide higher ratios of registered nurses to nonlicensed staff because some studies have been able to demonstrate a reduction of length of stay with higher nursing ratios.[10]
Efficient	Avoiding waste, including waste of equipment, supplies, ideas, and energy	Nurses are well known for their ability to work around obstacles to work around obstacles to get their patients access to necessary care and resources.[11] Along with their resourcefulness and willingness to navigate the system, nurses are well positioned to identify shortcomings of current processes. Unmistakably, the involvement of frontline nurses in quality improvement is a key source of evidence for hospitals striving to achieve Magnet Status.[12]
Equitable	Providing care that does not vary in quality because of personal characteristics, such as gender, ethnicity, geographic location, and socioeconomic status	The first provision of the Code of Ethics for Nurses as put forth by the American Nurses Association decrees that nurses practice with respect and compassion for each individual. "The nurse, in all professional relationships, practices with compassion and respect for the inherent dignity, worth, and uniqueness of every individual, unrestricted by considerations of social or economic status, personal attributes, or the nature of health problems." This provision is in accordance with the recommendation for patient-centered care because it acknowledges the importance of recognizing each individual, with special consideration to vulnerable populations, so that the clinical decisions made are consistent with what is considered the well-being for that particular individual.[13]

Adapted from Committee on Quality of Health Care in America, The Institute of Medicine. Crossing the quality chasm: a new health system for the 21st century. Washington, DC: National Academy Press; 2001. Reprinted with permission from the National Academies Press, Copyright © 2001 National Academy of Sciences.

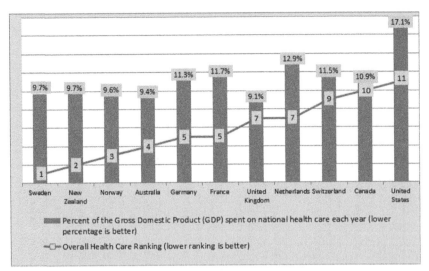

Fig. 1. United States is in the *highest* tier for expenditures, resulting in the highest cost. U.S. is also in the *highest* tier for Overall Health as defined by lower patient outcomes, lower quality, and lower efficiency. (*Total health expenditures data from* World Health Organization. Health expenditure, total (% of GDP). World Bank Group. 2015. Available at: http://data.worldbank.org/indicator/SH.XPD.TOTL.ZS. Accessed September 17, 2015; and *ranking data from* Davis K, Stremikis K, Squires D, et al. Mirror, mirror on the wall, 2014 update: how the performance of the U.S. health care system compares internationally. The Commonwealth Fund. Available at: http://www.commonwealthfund.org/publications/fund-reports/2014/jun/mirror-mirror. Accessed September 17, 2015.)

conditions as opposed to fatal diseases.[17] This phenomenon is increasingly evident throughout the lifespan (**Fig. 2**). Chronic conditions account for a majority of hospital admissions, prescriptions, and physician visits.[18]

POOR QUALITY OF CARE MAY PERPETUATE COSTS

With a growing number of persons with 1 or more chronic conditions, the oversight of care between subspecialties and multiple providers is essential to ensure that the patients have clinical and pharmacologic coordination.[18] The increase of chronic conditions, as well as an aging population, creates more stress on the primary care system. Additionally, there are a larger number of health consumers seeking care given the expansion of coverage under the Affordable Care Act. Primary care providers are already a scarce resource, especially in rural and underserved areas – unmistakably the same populations that have the highest incidence of chronic conditions.[19] Limitations to access create an environment where typically manageable chronic conditions progress, quality of care suffers, disease progresses, and costs perpetuate.

NURSES NAVIGATING AN EVOLVING ECONOMIC AND REGULATORY LANDSCAPE

Health insurance agencies must provide coverage to a larger number of consumers. In this landscape, reimbursement to health care organizations and providers is decreasing and payers are more frequently disputing charges. Health care organizations are challenged to identify how they can reduce internal cost and justify clinical care. The electronic health record, originally intended to improve the organization and flow of health information, has been used to account for evidence to meet

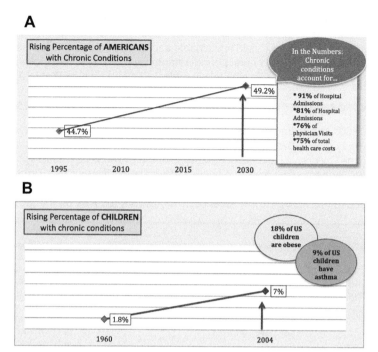

Fig. 2. Increasing percentages of the US population that live with at least one chronic illness. (*A*) Projected percentages of the US population that will be diagnosed with a chronic condition by the year 2030. (*B*) Rising percentage of US Children diagnosed with a chronic illness.

standards, such as with meaningful use.[20] The additional and sometimes duplicative work on the front line to capture care often falls on a bedside nurse, because current processes are not ideally positioned to reflect what is happening at the point of care.[21] External challenges of the health care environment often drive cost reduction exercises, leaving bedside nurse staffing less than optimal. Additionally, enhanced technology and complexity of patients all add a competition of priorities for bedside nurses and an ultimate list of intrinsic threats for nurses to address in daily work, while trying to assure safety and quality remain the top priority.

IMPORTANCE OF NURSE LEADERS DRIVING THE CULTURE OF A HIGH-RELIABILITY ORGANIZATION

To successfully overcome the challenges in the current environment, organizations must first empower frontline nurses to speak up and assure nurses are heard. Nurse leaders must be visible and aware of the problems within their areas. The importance of transparency and reporting on every near-miss event must be taken seriously. In return, senior leaders must be willing to take time to facilitate root cause analyses with frontline nursing staff, physicians, and leaders on serious and near-miss events to understand the problems and identify recommendations to prevent an event from occurring again. Staff at each level should be engaged and participative in these root cause analyses. It is imperative for nursing leadership to utilize a shared leadership model in an HRO, whereby staff is fully engaged and at the table for decision making.

An HRO creates an environment where adherence to evidence-based care is measured and shared. Commonly, nursing quality performance benchmarks hospital's outcomes against other like-hospitals. To elevate the commitment to patient safety and high quality, hospitals should place more emphasis on reliability to process measures, which will yield sustainable and uniform processes for the delivery of high-quality care. Through nurses' understanding of the HRO principles, leaders can educate staff on how each principle is critical to effect change (**Table 2**).

SOLUTIONS FOR PATIENT SAFETY: A UNIQUE OPPORTUNITY FOR PEDIATRICS

Since the 1980s, the children's hospitals in Ohio have shared a mission to reduce harmful events that occur within their institutions. Along with 25 children's hospitals across the nation, the Children's Hospital of Pittsburgh of the University of Pittsburgh Medical Center (CHP), accepted the opportunity to join the collaborative in 2011. The network of hospitals, now called Solutions for Patient Safety, has grown to include more than 80 children's hospitals across North America. The network focuses on the reduction of

Table 2 Manifestation of high-reliability organization principles in health care organizations		
Principle	**Nurses Can...**	**Leaders Can...**
Preoccupation with failure	Patient safety errors and near-miss events are readily reported by nurses. Nurses are not fearful to question and speak up when they have concerns.	Error reporting is encouraged and nonpunitive. Events and near misses are investigated with a systems approach. Information regarding apparent and root causes to events are freely shared to spread awareness.
Sensitivity to operations	Nurses are acutely aware of system and department risks to patient safety. Nurses have access to reliability and outcome measures. The definition of quality care is not limited to outcomes but incorporates performance.	Leaders invest resources to remove the barriers that prevent optimum performance. Leaders are well attuned to the threats and system shortcomings at the front line.
Reluctance to simplify interpretations	Nurses are comfortable providing honest, detailed information about near misses and events that reach patients. Nurses encourage fellow nurses to challenge current practice and raise concerns without judgment or the mentality of "this is the way it's always been done."	Leaders listen carefully; they trust and respect the input from frontline staff. Leaders create an environment that values skepticism and takes a strong stance against disrespect within all levels of the organization.
Commitment to resilience	Nurses learn from their mistakes; they ask "what if." They do not turn on themselves or others when events occur.	Leaders empower the front line to respond to and mitigate unexpected problems in real time. Leaders support staff that are involved in events.
Deference to expertise	Nurses are actively engaged in designing and implementing solutions. Nurses value their own expertise and confidently share their ideas.	Leaders include the individuals involved in events to identify root and apparent causes.

Adapted from Weick K, Sutcliffe K. Managing the unexpected: resilient performance in the age of uncertainty. 2nd edition. San Francisco: John Wiley &Sons, Inc; 2007.

10 hospital-acquired conditions (HACs) and the promotion of an organizational culture that promotes patient safety and quality. Each network hospital is charged to identify best practice bundles that, when followed, reduce the incidence of that particular HAC (**Table 3**). Furthermore, each hospital measures and submits their reliability to

Table 3
Monitoring reliability and outcomes related to hospital-acquired conditions

Hospital-Acquired Condition	Process Measure	Outcome Measure
Central line–associated blood stream infections	Insertion bundle: prevention measures for insertion of central lines Maintenance bundle: prevention measures for routine maintenance of central lines	Number of central line–associated blood stream infections per 1000 central line days
Catheter-associated urinary tract infections	Insertion bundle: prevention measures during Foley catheter insertion Maintenance bundle: prevention measures for patients with an indwelling Foley catheter	Number of catheter-associated urinary tract infections per 1000 Foley catheter days
Patient falls with injury	Prevention bundle: measures to prevent falls for all admitted patients	Number of falls that result in moderate or greater injury per 1000 patient days
Pressure ulcers	Prevention bundle: measures to prevent the development of pressure ulcers for all admitted patients	Number of pressure ulcers (stages 3 and 4 and unstageable)
Surgical site infections	Prevention bundle: measures preoperatively and intraoperatively that reduce infections at surgical sites	Number of surgical site infections per 100 cardiothoracic, neuroshunt, and spinal fusion cases
Readmissions	Discharge bundle: measures that reduce the likelihood that patients will be readmitted	Number of 7-day readmissions per 100 discharges
Ventilator-associated pneumonia	Prevention bundle: measures to prevent the prevalence of pneumonia in ventilated patients	Number of ventilated patients who acquire a ventilator per 1000 ventilator days
Venous thromboembolism events	Prevention bundle: measures that prevent the development of venous thrombosis	Number of venous thromboembolism events per 1000 patient days
Adverse drug events	Prevention bundle: measures that prevent the administration of the adverse drug events (ie, wrong dose, wrong route, wrong time, wrong patient, and/or wrong medication)	Number of adverse drug events (categories F–I on the the Medication Errors Reporting and Prevention scale) per 1000 patient days
Obstetric adverse events	Prevention bundle: measure that prevent serious obstetric harm events at network hospitals that have birthing units (CHP does not have a birthing center and, therefore, does not measure this HAC)	Number of obstetric events per 100 births

such bundles, emphasizing the importance of process measures, rather than solely focusing on outcomes. The transparent platform for network hospitals to freely share their internal prevention measures (bundles), their reliability to those bundles, their experiences and challenges, and their outcomes replaces the former environment of competition with collaboration and comradery to reduce harmful events to children and to improve the quality of care across all pediatric organizations.

FRONTLINE NURSES AND PHYSICIANS DRIVING SAFETY AND QUALITY TO REACH OUTCOMES

The responsibility of hospital leadership, as supported by the Institute of Medicine, is to provide an environment whereby nurses on the front line are involved in the strategy and implementation of work that improves quality and ensures patient safety. This is also identified as a key source of evidence for the designation of Magnet Recognition by the American Nurses Association. CHP intentionally partners nurses with physicians to colead individual HAC teams as well as the overarching Solutions for Patient Safety leadership dyad at the CHP. The collective transparency of reliability to prevention bundles on the national and local levels allows frontline staff in all network hospitals to actively participate in the work that affects their performance at the point of care. As a result, frontline nurses across the country become champions for quality improvement and patient safety. As a result of the collaborative physician and nurse-empowered leadership teams at CHP, there has been a 55% reduction in total number of serious safety events since the beginning of its participation in 2011 (**Fig. 3**).

The institute of Medicine Future of Nursing Report recommends that 80% of the nursing workforce in each health care organization should be baccalaureate (BSN) prepared by the year 2020. The recommendation was based on evidence which demonstrated that organizations with higher percentages of nurses with BSN degrees resulted in better patient outcomes including lower mortality rates, a decrease in failure to rescue rates, and a decrease in hospital acquired infections*. Significant efforts

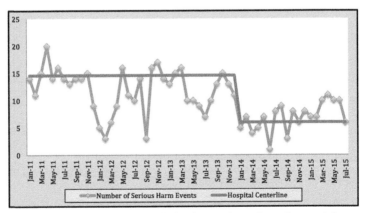

Fig. 3. CHP serious harm event data include the total number of central line–associated blood stream infections, catheter-associated urinary tract infections, ventilator-associated pneumonias, venous thromboembolism events, falls of moderate or greater harm, surgical site infections (cardiothoracic, neuroshunt, and spinal fusions), pressure ulcers (stages 3 and 4 and unstageable), and adverse drug events (F–I on the Medication Errors Reporting and Prevention scale).

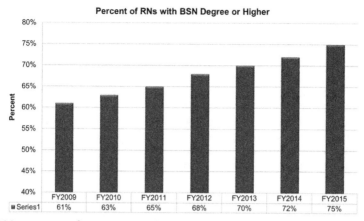

Fig. 4. Rising percent of RNs at CHP with a Baccalaureate Degree.

have been initiated at CHP to increase the number of employed BSN-prepared RNs, including recruitment strategies and support for current RNs returning to school (**Fig. 4**). CHP has demonstrated a 30% increase over the last eight years, and is expected to surpass their internal goal of having 90% of RNs with a BSN by the year 2020.

Similarly to the studies by Kelly and colleagues,[22] CHP has also observed a decrease in the rates of mortality as the percentage of RNs with a BSN have increased (**Fig. 5**).

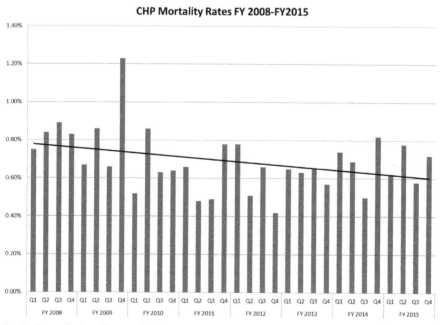

Fig. 5. Rate of Mortality at Children's Hospital of Pittsburgh of UPMC.

SUMMARY

The threats to quality care and patient safety are largely attributed to system, not human, errors. Leaders of health care organizations must be cognizant of the significant challenges that present to the frontline nursing staff. As the public and private expectations for quality increase, leaders must identify sustainable processes that yield positive patient outcomes, while at the same time aligning with the economic market, and that generate a positive work environment for nursing. As organizations strive for high quality, culture of safety, and greater efficiency while offering the best patient experience, nursing leaders must recognize the competitive priorities and filter safety and quality to the top of the list. As Nightingale said a century and a half ago, "The first requirement in a hospital is that it should do the sick no harm."

REFERENCES

1. American International Group (AIG), Inc. Patient safety; hospital risk – perspectives of hospital C-suite and risk managers. New York: 2013.
2. Becker Hospital Review. 11 Most Concerning Issues for Hospital CEOs. 2014. Available at: www.beckershospitalreview.com. Accessed September 17, 2015.
3. Nightingale F. Notes on nursing: what it is, and what it is not. First American edition. New York: D. Appleton and Company; 1860. Available at: http://digital.library.upenn.edu/women/nightingale/nursing/nursing.html.
4. The Institute of Medicine. To err is human: building a safer health system. Washington, DC: National Academy Press; 1999. Available at: http://iom.nationalacademies.org/~/media/Files/Report%20Files/1999/To-Err-is-Human/To%20Err%20is%20Human%201999%20%20report%20brief.pdf. Accessed September 17, 2015.
5. The Institute of Medicine. Crossing the quality chasm: a new health system for the 21st century. Washington, DC: National Academy Press; 2001.
6. Gaylord GP. Nursing advocacy: an ethic of practice. Nurs Ethics 1995;2(1):11–8.
7. Su-yin H, Godbold N, Collier A, et al. Finding the patient in patient safety. Broadway, Sydney (Australia): Centre for Health Communication, University of Technology; 2013.
8. Pipe TB, Wellik KE, Buchda VL, et al. Implementing evidence-based nursing practice. Urol Nurs 2005;25(5):365–70. Available at: http://www.medscape.com/viewarticle/514532.
9. Kuo DZ, Houtrow AM, Arango P, et al. Family-centered care: Current applications and future directions in pediatric health care. Maternal and Child Health Journal 2012;16(2):297–305.
10. Thungjaroenkul P, Cummings GG, Embleton A. The impact of nurse staffing on hospital costs and patient length of stay: a systematic review. Nurs Econ 2007;25(5):255–65.
11. Ebright PR, Patterson ES, Chalko BA, et al. Understanding the complexity of registered nurse work in acute care settings. J Nurs Adm 2003;33(12):630–8.
12. Needleman J, Hassmiller S. The role of nurses in improving hospital quality and efficiency: real-world results. Health Aff 2009;28(4):625–33.
13. Fowler MDM. Guide to the code of ethics for nurses: interpretation and application. Silver Spring (MD): American Nurses Association; 2010. Available at: http://www.nursesbooks.org/ebooks/download/CodeofEthics.pdf.
14. World Health Organization. Health expenditure, total (% of GDP). World Bank Group. 2015. Available at: http://data.worldbank.org/indicator/SH.XPD.TOTL.ZS. Accessed September 17, 2015.

15. Davis K, Stremikis K, Squires D, et al. Mirror, mirror on the wall, 2014 update: how the performance of the U.S. health care system compares internationally. The Commonwealth Fund. Available at: http://www.commonwealthfund.org/publications/fund-reports/2014/jun/mirror-mirror. Accessed September 17, 2015.
16. Centers for Medicare & Medicaid Services. National health expenditure projections 2014. 2024. Office of the Actuary, National Health Statistics Group. Available at: https://www.cms.gov/Research-Statistics-Data-and-Systems/Statistics-Trends-and-Reports/NationalHealthExpendData/Downloads/proj2014.pdf. Accessed September 17, 2015.
17. Rothman AA, Wagner EH. Chronic illness management: what is the role of primary care? Ann Intern Med 2003;138(3):256–61.
18. Partnership for Solutions. Chronic conditions: making the case for ongoing care. September 2004 Update. Available at: http://www.rwjf.org/files/research/chronic%20conditions%20Chartbook@209-2004ppt. Accessed September 17, 2015.
19. Ward BW, Clarke TC, Freeman G, et al. Early release of selected estimates based on data for the 2014 national health interview survey. Division of Health Interview Statistics, National Center for Health Statistics; 2015. Available at: http://www.cdc.gov/nchs/data/nhis/earlyrelease/earlyrelease201506.pdf.
20. EHR Incentives & Certification. 2013. HealthIT.gov. Available at: https://www.healthit.gov/providers-professionals/ehr-incentives-certification. Accessed September 17, 2015.
21. Stokowski LA. Electronic nursing documentation: charting new territory. Medscape Nurses. 2013. Available at: http://www.medscape.com/viewarticle/810573_5. Accessed September 17, 2015.
22. Kelly LA, McHugh MD, Aiken LH. Nurse outcomes in Magnet and non-magnet hospitals. Journal Nursing Administration 2011;41(10):428–33.

Pediatric Quality Improvement

Practical and Scholarly Considerations

Matthew F. Niedner, MD

KEYWORDS

- Quality improvement • Patient safety • Medical errors • Implementation science
- Translational research

KEY POINTS

- This article describes important aspects of health-care quality, quality improvement, patient safety, and how to do research on efforts to improve performance in the delivery of health care.
- The case for improving health care quality is outlined, with an emphasis on the special considerations within the pediatric setting.
- Common terminology to facilitate an understanding of quality is reviewed, including near-misses, and preventable and nonpreventable adverse events.
- Models for understanding system and process performance are discussed, including the system of profound knowledge, aims-oriented change and plan-do-study-act applications of the scientific method.

WHAT IS HEALTH-CARE QUALITY?

In *To Err Is Human*, the Institute of Medicine (IOM) defined health-care quality as "the degree to which health services increase the likelihood of desired outcomes" and patient safety (PS) as "freedom from accidental injury because of medical care or medical errors."[1] These two concepts are fundamentally linked, and many notable authorities have explicitly cited safety as the key dimension of quality, including the IOM, the Leapfrog Group, the Institute for Healthcare Improvement (IHI), the National Quality Forum, and even Hippocrates: primum non nocere. In this article, quality improvement (QI) is used as a broad term that encompasses not only enhanced positive performance but also mitigation or elimination of errors, health care defects, and patient harm.

Pediatric Intensive Care Unit, Division of Critical Care Medicine, Department of Pediatrics, Mott Children's Hospital, University of Michigan Medical Center, F-6894 Mott #0243, 1500 East Medical Center Drive, Ann Arbor, MI 48109-0243, USA
E-mail address: mniedner@med.umich.edu

Pediatr Clin N Am 63 (2016) 341–356
http://dx.doi.org/10.1016/j.pcl.2015.12.006
0031-3955/16/$ – see front matter Published by Elsevier Inc.

pediatric.theclinics.com

The IOM's *Crossing the Quality Chasm* outlined 6 dimensions of health-care quality.[2] The most fundamental attribute is that care should be safe. Care must also be effective and appropriately dispensed, avoiding underuse and overuse by being provided to all who could benefit and not to those unlikely to benefit. Care should be patient centered; respectful of and responsive to individual patient preferences, needs, and values. Quality care is timely; the right care to the right person at the right time, with waits and delays eliminated or minimized. Care should be efficient, actively seeking to identify and eliminate all forms of waste, be it time, equipment, supplies, or energy. The final dimension of care outlined by the IOM is equitability: the provision of care that does not vary in quality because of personal characteristics such as sex, ethnicity, geographic location, and socioeconomic status. In "Revisiting the Quality Chasm", Brilli and colleagues[3] reorganized these same IOM dimensions in a patient-centric framework as follows: do not harm me, cure me, treat me with respect, navigate my care, and keep us well. Strategies used to apply evidence to achieve these missions are largely the domain of QI. QI research is the rigorous analysis of what makes QI efforts effective, sustainable, worth the investment, or vice versa.

QUALITY IMPROVEMENT, RESEARCH, AND QUALITY IMPROVEMENT RESEARCH

It is common for classic research and QI interventions to be confused, because they both are seeking to improve patient outcomes in data-driven ways, although typically through different mechanisms. Classic research in early translational stages often defines the best known practices that QI agents strive to implement in later translational work. However, improvements in the performance reliability of baseline clinical practices can reduce noise, improving the sensitivity of analyses designed to detect small incremental improvements in best practice. If children are not afflicted by preventable nosocomial infections, medication errors, or surgical complications, then sensitivity is improved when trying to detect the impact of a novel research intervention on patient outcomes.

This blurred boundary between classic research and QI is well recognized, and derives from the intent of both to result in better outcomes for patients, albeit with a different perspective, through different methodologies, and tolerating different thresholds for risk.[4] This is particularly true for T3 translational research regarding either the operationalization of established best practice or adoption of general principles such as standardization to uniform common practice. Because many peer-review journals require formal institutional review board comment on approval or exemption, many QI/PS projects focused on organizational and operational performance simply go unreported. However, scholarly work in QI/PS has been published with year-on-year increases since the IOM's 1999 publication of *To Err Is Human*.[2] Because of the increasing scholarly output in this area of medicine, both in quantity and quality, the expectations for the quality of QI research are also steadily mounting. Calls for scholarly accounts of quality and safety endeavors, along with publication guidelines for proper peer review, have appeared in recent years.[5,6] Notably, the strengths and weaknesses of the Standards for Quality Improvement Reporting Excellence (SQUIRE) guidelines of 2008 have undergone critical review with updated 2015 guidelines to provide better planning and publication guidance for QI researchers.[7] Many of the methodologies to analyze quality and safety in health care with academic rigor are still in development, young, and under adaptation from other industries and disciplines, and many are neither familiar to practicing clinicians nor embedded in medical education.[8] Such analytical tools from human-factors engineering, psychology, industrial engineering, and manufacturing are increasingly being accepted in the traditional peer-reviewed medical literature.[9]

Perhaps one of the simplest ways to think of QI is as a strategy to close the gap between actual practice and best known practice, be it clinical or operational.[10] The estimated lag time for scientific knowledge generated in randomized clinical trials to be routinely accepted into medical practice is 17 years; a shocking testimony to the size and persistence of the gap between the evidence and actual care, and a provocative invitation to close it.[2] **Fig. 1** shows how QI fits in the context of actual, best, and idealized performance. If the graph is taken as a survival or time-to-adverse-event curve from some identified measure of quality or safety, it can be assumed that the ideal outcome is 100% perfect over time. Much conventional research is focused on closing the gap between current best practice and such an idealized practice; that is, taking the best known mousetrap and incrementally making it better. In contrast, much QI is focused on closing the gap between actual practice and best known practice; that is, taking the best-designed mousetrap already known and ensuring that it deploys flawlessly every time it is indicated (and not when it is not) in the specific local context of deployment.[11]

Health services research (HSR), like classic research, can inform interventional QI efforts, but HSR is typically passive, often taking advantage of natural experiments; it analyzes differences in outcomes based on variations in context or care delivery that already exist instead of implementing practice changes to optimize outcomes.

Unlike clinically or physiologically oriented classic research, HSR studies often incorporate how social factors, organizational structures, delivery processes, financial drivers, and personal behaviors affect health-care access, quality, cost, and outcomes.[12] HSR methodologies, data management, and statistical approaches often draw on the same biostatistical traditions of clinical research. HSR often shows where improvement could or should occur in health care and the degree to which improvement might affect outcomes, and even suggests the factors that may be essential targets for change. HSR may be considered a form of early QI research in terms of informing QI interventions, but it is distinct from the analysis or research performed on interventions undertaken to improve quality. The research methods commonly used to analyze QI interventions are distinct from both traditional research and HSR.

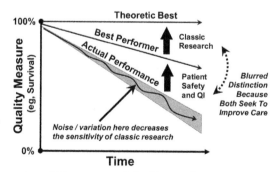

Fig. 1. Classic research and QI are synergistic drivers of improvement. Classic prospective interventional research and QI both seek to move clinical care closer to an idealized theoretic best outcome. Classic research often focuses on novel means, such as more sensitive diagnostics or superior therapeutics. QI often focuses on closing the gap between common practice and established best practice, such as through standardization, decision support, and automation. Reducing errors and performance variation in operations through QI can reduce the noise introduced into measures of research interest, thereby improving the sensitivity of research efforts. Thus, clinical research and clinical QI are synergistic.

The term translational research encompasses a long sequence of analysis from bench to bedside to practice guidelines. Research guided primarily by physiologic principles occurs in the early stages of translational research (ie, T1 and T2). However, unlike early translational research, late translational research (ie, T3), such as implementation science, performance reliability, or improvement sustainability, is often profoundly influenced by local phenomena (eg, staffing ratios, case mix), individualism (eg, clinicians' experience base, leadership styles), human factors (eg, psychology, ergonomics), and nonmedical forces (eg, business plans, economics, information technology, industrial engineering). These types of factors often affect the ability to generalize many local or single-site quality and safety interventions, so their inclusion in the analytical plan of QI research is often of utmost importance. As center after center tragically reinvent the wheel locally, most discoveries from T3 translational activity are never published or disseminated in a scholarly manner; a lost opportunity in terms of the knowledge that can be extracted.[13]

In summary, research is the discovery of new knowledge and evidence on which clinicians can base their practices, QI is work designed to deliver the best possible evidence-based care consistently in local contexts, and QI research is the rigorous analysis of the improvement or implementation of the work itself. The clinical or operational outcomes of QI work are a barometer of the effectiveness of the QI intervention, but QI research strives to establish the viability of aims, the appropriateness of scope, the efficacy of change methods used, the interdependent array of results beyond primary outcomes (including process and balancing measures), and the influence of contextual factors either facilitating or impeding improvement efforts. Such clinical QI research produces, at one level, replication studies of primary evidence, but more importantly it creates insights into what contributed to effective or ineffective implementation work in real-world and often diverse settings, allowing others to generalize these insights and either emulate successes or anticipate potential pitfalls when attempting to apply the same evidence.

MODELS FOR UNDERSTANDING QUALITY

As experimental statistician George Box[14] observed, "All models are wrong, but some are useful." Models provide an artificial structure for knowledge that reflects complex phenomena accurately enough to better enable understanding; ideally well enough to enable meaningful interpretation and informed action. Health-care quality is complex, but models can help clinicians to grasp what is essential. Beyond organizing QI work, these models can also serve as the organizational framework for QI research. A few of the more common and useful models for improvement are touched on here.

A common mode for organizing quality and safety analyses relates to the hierarchy of defects in a complex system. Latent system risks, near-misses, and actual harm are points along a continuum. **Fig. 2** shows how this continuum matches the QI methods commonly used to remediate such defects. There is a long-standing debate about whether it is more advantageous to measure risk, errors, or harm, but, in truth, each has advantages and disadvantages, and all are widely used.

Detection and elimination of latent defects in a complex system provides the ideal solution to improving quality and safety, because it is the furthest point upstream from harming a patient. Failure modes and effects analysis (FMEA) is a powerful strategy to identify ways in which a complex system can fail because of the known historical performance of constituent parts of a device or process. This strategy allows potential defects to be designed out of the system (or planned countermeasures to be devised)

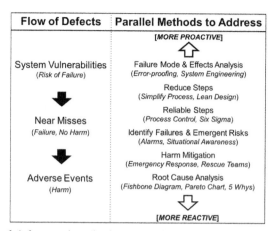

Fig. 2. Hierarchy of defects and methods to remediate.

before a design culminates in a product or an active process. FMEA is widely used in manufacturing and engineering industries in which device performance is fairly predictable (as with an intravenous pump or telemetry unit), but it is increasingly applied in the service industry.[15] Limitations of analyzing latent system vulnerabilities include a lack of good historical performance data on which to base the model; the risk of unforeseen perturbations in complex and interdependent systems; unpredictable and dynamic changes in the system; lack of intuitive guidance to the sources of risk; and the theoretic nature of some assumptions and conclusions in the absence of measurable errors or harm.

Another top-tier tool in system improvement is process streamlining through the elimination of waste, be it time, energy, materials, or process complexity. Albert Einstein is quoted as saying, "Make everything as simple as possible, but not simpler."[16] If a desired outcome can be achieved in fewer steps without loss of fidelity or performance, it is likely to be more reliable, because eliminating unnecessary steps removes some opportunities for errors to creep into a system and simultaneously reduces the number of variables when trying to understand ongoing failures. Furthermore, elimination of waste improves value from a cost-benefit perspective. This kind of streamlining to optimize value-added output is the basis for lean design, originally applied to production lines but increasingly applied to service lines. The contemporary paradigm of lean production and management is based on the Toyota Production System, and lean strategies have been successfully adapted to health care.[17–19] A full description of lean methodology is beyond the scope of this article, but exhaustive resources are available for interested students.[20,21]

Progressing along the ladder from latent defect to harm, the next step includes errors. A widely accepted definition for medical error is failure of a planned action to be completed as intended (an error of execution) or the use of a wrong plan to achieve an aim (an error of planning), whether by commission or omission.[22] Thus the drug overdose caused by a decimal error may be considered an error of execution by commission, whereas the treatment of mistaken septic shock instead of the actual adrenal crisis might be viewed as an error of planning in which proper care was omitted. If the error results in no harm, it is commonly labeled a near-miss, whereas if harm occurs it is considered a preventable adverse event. This situation should be considered distinct from nonpreventable adverse events for which ways to avoid the known complication are not established; that is, harm occurring as a consequence of medical care but in the absence of an error (such as with the risk of cardiotoxicity from certain chemotherapeutic agents). Because errors resulting in near-misses are far more common than errors resulting in preventable harm, near-misses provide an attractive target for monitoring and measuring quality and safety on a continuous basis. Analysis of near-misses in an iterative manner can help generate hypotheses for root causes more rapidly than if only harmful events are considered. Focusing on errors can be particularly helpful when related outcome measures are too rare or catastrophic to be acceptable guides (eg, deaths). Such error-based surveillance (eg, compliance with a best practice) is particularly helpful when there is good evidence for key steps or processes firmly established in the medical literature. The ability to identify and monitor compliance with important process measures provides actionable data to an improvement team about how to reduce unnecessary variation and close the gap between actual performance and desired best practice. This ability is the basis of process control, and is often associated with the Six Sigma management strategy used widely in many sectors of industry, including health care.

Although there are advantages to error-based quality-performance analyses, there are notable limitations to acknowledge. Error and near-miss rates vary widely depending on the definitions used for error, the surveillance methods, and even the safety culture of the reporting unit, which confounds the external validity of such quantification.[23,24] Measures of errors are most helpful if they can be expressed as rates (errors divided by opportunities for that error type), but there is no denominator available for many types of error and harm.[25] Even the numerators can be circumspect because many errors go unreported, and there is an attention bias that favors identification of errors of commission (rather than omission) and errors resulting in harm (rather than near-misses).[26] Data derived from voluntary error reporting are particularly messy. In a survey of pediatric physicians and nurses, half filed incident reports on less than 50% of their own errors, and a third did so less than 20% of the time.[26] It is reasonable to conclude that most practitioners are only aware of the tip of the iceberg when it comes to near-misses, preventable harm, and opportunities for improving health-care quality. Thus, error-based quality assessment may be better applied as a local qualitative and semiquantitative improvement strategy, rather than an as a comparative performance tool.[27]

The measure of actual harm to patients is a final measure of quality and safety in the current hierarchy being discussed. From a high-principled perspective, harm to the patient can be considered a failure to detect and mitigate the latent system defects and combination of conspiring errors or contexts. This situation is often described as the Swiss -cheese model, whereby an error or errors propagate through a system that is designed to intercept such errors but that, because of system dynamism and complexity, does not prevent all harm from reaching a patient.[28] Although risk and near-miss analyses are more proactive, harm analysis is a more reactive process; there is no putting the genie back in the bottle. However, from a pragmatic perspective it is adding insult to injury to witness harm and not try to learn from it. It is worth noting that all errors are not equal; those resulting in harm may be distinct from those that do not, and harmful errors can implicate defects not necessarily apparent in near-misses.[29]

Several organizations have proposed injury-based trigger tools that can be used to provide systematic surveillance measures of harm, such as the Agency for Healthcare Research and Quality's general and pediatric-specific PS indicators, the IHI's Global Trigger Tool, and others.[25,30–33] Some of these metrics and tools focus on types of harm that are assumed to be preventable or largely so, whereas other tools for measuring harm are inclusive of all readily identifiable harm. One key advantage to measuring all harm is that it provides an opportunity to question the boundary between preventable and unpreventable injuries. If the goal in health care is to eliminate or reduce all harm to patients, then including measures of harm considered unpreventable by traditional medical standards can direct clinicians' attention toward innovative care or research. It is the medical legacy that types of harm formerly deemed to be a cost of doing business are now considered largely preventable.[34–36]

Harm-based performance metrics have their limitations too, the most obvious being that the patient is injured in some manner. Because unpreventable adverse events and deaths are, to some extent, expected in hospital settings, such occurrences do not necessarily raise the specter of preventable error. When they are recognized, attribution may not be accurate. Furthermore, the retrospective nature of harm evaluation provokes numerous kinds of bias toward which human perceptions are prone, such as hindsight and outcome bias.[37] If the analysis and attribution of risk, error, or harm are significantly biased, incorrect, or overly simplistic, then the conclusions not only are invalid but also can lead to unnecessary and possibly counterproductive attempts at remediation. Therefore, all risk, error, and harm analysis, as well as planned responses, must be undertaken with such limits and pitfalls in mind. In addition, because all monitoring and corrective strategies have limitations and none are perfectly suited for all applications, it makes sense to use multiple simultaneous approaches for a more robust quality-monitoring and safety-monitoring system. Doing so also helps create cross-validation between sources of perceived risks, error patterns, and actual harm, helping to overcome the weaknesses of each individual approach.

THE SCIENCE OF QUALITY IMPROVEMENT

When considering QI science, especially late translational research, an understanding of the realistic evaluation model put forward by Pawson and Tilley[38] is helpful to get past some of the constraints inherent in orthodox experimentation.[39] Realistic evaluation seeks to explain variation in outcomes by analyzing the context that may have differentially enabled or disabled an intervention from having the postulated impact. Classic research methods use strategies to wash out variation and isolate the effect of an intervention, such as with randomization, prospective analysis, large sample sizes, blinding, and controlling for known confounders. If the literature is conflicted on the efficacy of an intervention, a conventional approach might be to perform a meta-analysis, essentially to group the studies together to see what the true effect is when analyzed with greater power. However compellingly large the sample size may become, there are many limitations to this method of understanding variation between studies.[40–42] Another way to interpret conflicting studies is to consider the unknown, unmeasured, or unrecognized contextual factors that altered the impact of an intervention (either positively or negatively) in different studies or sites. If influential contextual factors can be identified, implementing such enablers or eliminating disablers may allow an intervention to perform as intended. A good example of this is the impact of safety culture on certain unit outcomes, such as nosocomial infection rates, throughput delays, medication errors, and staff turnover.[43–47] Teamwork and safety climate have proved to be responsive to local interventions, both positively and negatively, making interventional anthropology a growing domain of QI.[44,48]

Not only are the models for QI science often different from traditional biostatistical approaches, but the way measures are viewed and used also differ (**Table 1**).[49,50]

Table 1
Comparison of measures in classic research versus QI science

	Classic Research	Improvement/Safety Science
Usual goals	Discovery of new knowledge; providing objective proof or basis; establishing best practice	Operationalize discoveries or best practice into routine care; ensure/monitor performance
Intervention or protocol	Single static protocol; first and last patient in protocol get same management; long timetables	Flexible/dynamic protocol or multiple serial tests; management adjusted freely based on learning; short and responsive timetables
Management of confounders	Identify, eliminate, exclude, and control for biases through blinding, randomization, crossover, and so forth	Identify and understand biases; stabilize biases during tests or interpret findings in bias context
Preferred measures	Hard and unequivocal outcomes; background data to ensure comparability	Blend of outcomes measures, relevant process measures, and possible balancing measures
Power and scale	Powered to definitively answer question and possibly explore post hoc analyses	Minimally sufficient data to meet confidence threshold for action or decision; successful tests scale up
Data interpretation	Data blinding; no interim peeking; data safety–monitoring boards; classic biostatistics with significance thresholds	Real-time data; analyze and act on data simultaneously; statistical process control (control charts); data trends influence next steps

Data from Solberg LI, Mosser G, McDonald S. The three faces of performance measurement: improvement, accountability, and research. Jt Comm J Qual Improv 1997;23:135–47; and Lloyd RC. In God we trust; all others bring data. Front Health Serv Manage 2007;23:33–8; [discussion: 43–5].

Classic research seeks to discover new knowledge in the scientific realm, whereas improvement science seeks to operationalize knowledge in real life. In research orthodoxy, unequivocal hard outcomes (eg, death) are preferable to surrogate markers assumed to be correlated with them (eg, multiple organ dysfunction scores). However, measures in improvement science are multidimensional, often with a hard outcome measure as an ultimate verification that improvement is occurring, but critically important process measures that serve as the tools to guide the specific improvement strategies used. An important example of the difference between QI process measures and traditional surrogate measures can be found in hand hygiene compliance. Although the hard outcome measure of hospital-acquired infections (HAIs) can be measured, it is hoped that they are infrequent events and do not lend themselves to rapidly determining efficacy of interventions to reduce them. However, hand hygiene compliance can be measured frequently, and rapid-cycle improvement interventions can be built around such key processes contributing to HAIs without waiting for adverse events to occur, and also without having to reprove germ theory with every QI intervention.

Classic research strives to have a rigorously consistent management protocol, whereas improvement science constantly tweaks and refines management toward best practice. Although classic research seeks to eliminate or minimize biases, improvement scientists try to hold known biases sufficiently steady during testing to allow for causal inference. Classic research is typically powered a priori to definitively answer a primary question with statistical significance once all the data are gathered, and interim analyses are shunned to avoid spurious signals. In contrast, improvement science seeks to generate real-time and continuous data that can be interpreted and acted on simultaneously, sometimes using data trends to inform confidence in recent interventions and guide the next steps from a probabilistic vantage point. For instance, if a QI intervention is inexpensive, safe, and minimally burdensome (eg, a central-line insertion checklist), then clinicians might accept a different level of confidence in the statistical significance of local implementation than, for example, if they were considering an intervention that is expensive, cumbersome, and accompanied by potential unintended consequences (eg, immunotherapy).

A large historical body of QI efforts is, in the eyes of many scientists, mere administrative window dressing; the rewriting of policies, the aesthetic revision of a patient portal Web site, the feel-good effects of patient-centered or family centered niceties.[47] However, the modern PS movement represents a sustained effort to use rigorous methods driven by data and testing. At the core of science, be it classic research or QI, is the scientific method. There are many ways to apply the scientific method, and the crucial challenge is to have sufficient knowledge of the tools and methods, to grasp their limitations, and to know which tool is appropriate for a particular problem at hand.[8,50,51] To this end, pioneers in the science of improvement have put forward an archetypal model for improvement that can serve as a fairly universal platform well suited for improvement work in health care.[52,53]

The model for improvement begins with a clear expression of aims in measurable and time-specific terms as applied to a defined population. As the IHI's motto goes, "Soon is not a time, some is not a number." The model for improvement calls for clearly defining or developing new metrics to track progress toward the aim in quantitative ways; some combination of outcome, process, and balancing measures to know whether improvement is taking place independent of subjective opinion. The crucial judgment step in this model is selecting the change to test. All improvement requires making changes, but not all changes result in improvement. Reliance on individuals with keen insight into the system complexities at hand as well as the operational realities is most helpful at this decision point, because an improvement team ideally selects from a host of possible changes the ones most likely to result in desirable change.

Once a candidate change is identified, the testing process can begin within the plan-do-study-act (PDSA) cycles. The PDSA structure is simply a bare-bones expression of the scientific method as it is applied in the work setting. PDSA is a decades-old construct offered by William Edwards Deming, PhD, and is analogous to the Six Sigma terminology for the scientific method as applied to process control; namely, define, measure, analyze, improve, control.[54] The PDSA approach is not intended as a one-off pilot study, but as an iterative, rapid-cycle, action-oriented learning approach without necessarily waiting for complete stabilization of effect before another PDSA is undertaken. This is a key difference between classic research with a protocolized intervention and QI, in which the intervention evolves in an iterative way over time.

How to determine the scope of PDSA work can be challenging, especially because some particularly vexing quality issues are difficult to fix in a piecemeal manner and may require system reengineering at a high level, such as through value stream mapping and lean redesign. However, much QI work can begin at a level suited to the confidence in change, the readiness of staff, and the costs of failure. PDSA cycles that fail to meet hypotheses should be scrutinized for reasons, whereas PDSA cycles that suggest or result in clear improvement should be considered for refinement and scaling up. Therefore, all PDSA cycles should generate learning. Failed PDSA cycles can often teach improvement teams more about a system than successful PDSA cycles because they can reveal faulty assumptions or important unrecognized variables.

STATISTICAL METHODS IN QUALITY IMPROVEMENT RESEARCH AND A PRIMER IN STATISTICAL PROCESS CONTROL

Various types of problems addressed by health-care improvement efforts may make certain types of solutions more or less effective. Not every problem can be solved with 1 QI method, but a problem often suggests its own best solution strategy. Similarly, the analytical strategy described in QI research should align with the rationale, project aims, and data constraints. Many approaches are available to help analyze health-care improvement, including qualitative approaches (eg, fishbone diagrams in root cause analysis, structured interviews with patients/families, gemba walks) or quantitative approaches (eg, interrupted time series analysis, traditional parametric and nonparametric testing between subgroups, logistic regression). Often the most effective analytical approach occurs when quantitative and qualitative data are clearly linked.

It is crucial for QI teams and researchers to understand variation in data to avoid making errors in interpretation. However, in practice, many QI teams do not have sufficient biostatistical training to have confidence in real-time interpretation of continuous data streams generated by their efforts. Although traditional biostatistical methods (eg, interrupted time series) can be used, this can stymie aims-oriented, data-driven, rapid-cycle PDSA improvement work. One accessible solution to this dilemma is for improvement teams to develop a working knowledge of statistical process control (SPC).[55–57] The basic component of SPC is the control chart, which serves as a graphical heuristic. It is not a hypothesis test but is constructed to generate insights into temporal signals in a complex system under a wide range of unknowable circumstances.

To grasp the essence of a control chart, imagine a conventional bell-shaped curve turned 90° on its side to give a horizontal set of lines corresponding with the mean and standard deviations (left pane of **Fig. 3**). Time is represented on the x-axis, and the performance metric on the y-axis. Sigma is similar to standard deviation, but depends on the type of control chart being used and is generally more sensitive in detecting significant outlying data. The plus and minus 3-sigma boundaries are called the upper and lower control limits, respectively. Accepting distributions of data within plus or minus 3 sigma of the mean (ie, within a total range of 6 sigma) affords a rational way to minimize type I and type II errors. When data are outside this range or show certain patterns, the system is considered out of control; that is, they lack consistent conformity to a central tendency.

Unlike a bell-shaped curve, in which data are collapsed into intervention versus control or preintervention versus postintervention categories, a control chart plots data over the axis of time (center pane of **Fig. 3**), providing insight into signals that emerge from the sequence of data measurements. The practical power of SPC is that people who are not statisticians can bring significant statistical rigor to their quantitative data in an intuitive format by understanding just a few simple, pattern-based rules to distinguish special-cause variation (ie, signals) from common-cause variation (ie, noise) (right pane of **Fig. 3**). These rules are fairly intuitive for anyone with a basic grasp of probabilities. For instance, any single data point more than 3 sigma (roughly equivalent to 3 standard deviations) from the mean should stand out as a signal for which an attributable cause should be sought, as should a series of 9 points on the same side of the mean line, which is tantamount to flipping 9 consecutive heads with a coin.

SPC is rooted in venerated time series analysis and is an available function in most advanced biostatistical software packages. However, such data can be readily maintained in simple spreadsheets, typically by entering numerators and denominators on

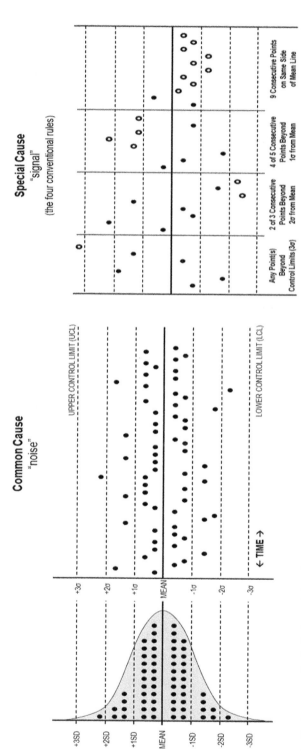

Fig. 3. Analogy of a bell-shaped distribution to control chart data and conventional rules for special cause.

whatever data-collection cycle is appropriate (eg, weekly, monthly, quarterly). This method allows QI teams to collect, interpret, and act on data in real-time, without the bottleneck created by relying on a statistician to intermittently decipher signals and noise. Some expertise is required in selecting the correct type of control chart when getting started, because, just as with traditional biostatistics, the nature of the measure (eg, continuous, integer, categorical) determines the proper control chart to use, although one control chart looks much the same as the next. For QI researchers, there are many analytical tools that can be used, both quantitative and qualitative. A thorough review of all conceivable methodologies is beyond the scope of this article. However, SPC is highlighted here because, although it is not routinely taught in biomedical statistics, it is a rigorous and pragmatic approach for both the QI work and the data analysis in scholarly manuscripts.

SUMMARY

At no other time have health-care quality and PS recognition been of greater import than they are now. The modern PS movement continues to grow at an unprecedented pace, both at pragmatic and academic levels. Pediatrics is an environment rich with the potential for risk, error, and harm. It is also full of dedicated, bright, vigilant people who have a wealth of clinical and operational information at their fingertips. This situation creates a very fertile environment to be able to engage in and pioneer QI science. Through PS work, pediatricians across the United States have reported successful reductions in central-line infections, ventilator-associated pneumonias, harmful medication errors, preventable asthma acute care visits, out-of-ICU cardiopulmonary arrests, and many other undesirable outcomes.[36,48,58–60] Through QI work, pediatricians have also disseminated knowledge of how to successfully improve vaccination rates, hand hygiene compliance, sepsis mortality, and multiorgan outcomes in chronic diseases, and myriad other opportunities.[61–64] The sustainability and spread of such improvements have historically proved patchy, but drivers are increasingly being understood.[65–67] Numerous examples of successful, pediatric-specific, multicenter QI collaboratives now exist as exemplars for operating at scale, which is important for both the clinical and academic dimensions of such work.[68]

Ingredients essential for QI and QI research to flourish are (1) local expertise in effective implementation science, (2) leaders committed and willing to resource a QI vision, (3) time and engagement of frontline staff members to execute such a vision, (4) a scholarly skill set to transform the QI work into credible knowledge that can be generalized, and (5) establishment of or engagement with networks of individuals and institutions to be able to execute QI and QI research at scale. This article outlines principles and approaches that should prove useful to clinicians rising to meet these challenges.

REFERENCES

1. Kohn LT, Corrigan J, Donaldson MS. To err is human: building a safer health system. Washington, DC: National Academy Press; 2000.
2. Institute of Medicine (US). Committee on Quality of Health Care in America. Crossing the quality chasm: a new health system for the 21st century. Washington, DC: National Academy Press; 2001.
3. Brilli RJ, Allen S, Davis JT. Revisiting the quality chasm. Pediatrics 2014;133: 763–5.
4. Morris PE, Dracup K. Quality improvement or research? The ethics of hospital project oversight. Am J Crit Care 2007;16:424–6.

5. Davidoff F, Batalden P, Stevens D, et al. Publication guidelines for quality improvement in health care: evolution of the SQUIRE project. Qual Saf Health Care 2008;17(Suppl 1):i3–9.
6. Speroff T, James BC, Nelson EC, et al. Guidelines for appraisal and publication of PDSA quality improvement. Qual Manag Health Care 2004;13:33–9.
7. Ogrinc G, Davies L, Goodman D, et al. SQUIRE 2.0 (Standards for QUality Improvement Reporting Excellence): revised publication guidelines from a detailed consensus process. BMJ Qual Saf; 2015.
8. Berwick DM. The science of improvement. JAMA 2008;299:1182–4.
9. Reason JT. The human contribution: unsafe acts, accidents and heroic recoveries. Farnham (United Kingdom); Burlington (VT): Ashgate; 2008.
10. Shojania KG, Ranji SR, Shaw LK, et al. Closing the Quality Gap: A Critical Analysis of Quality Improvement Strategies (Vol. 2: Diabetes Care). Rockville (MD): Agency for Healthcare Research and Quality; 2004.
11. Ting HH, Shojania KG, Montori VM, et al. Quality improvement: science and action. Circulation 2009;119:1962–74.
12. Sheikh K, Gilson L, Agyepong IA, et al. Building the field of health policy and systems research: framing the questions. PLoS Med 2011;8:e1001073.
13. Audet AM, Doty MM, Shamasdin J, et al. Measure, learn, and improve: physicians' involvement in quality improvement. Health Aff (Millwood) 2005;24:843–53.
14. Box GEP. Robustness in the strategy of scientific model building. In: Robustness in statistics. New York: Academic Press; 1979. p. 201–36.
15. Donchin Y, Gopher D, Olin M, et al. A look into the nature and causes of human errors in the intensive care unit. Crit Care Med 1995;23:294–300.
16. Sessions R. How a 'difficult' composer gets that way. New York Times 1950;1950. Sect. 89.
17. Jimmerson C, Weber D, Sobek DK 2nd. Reducing waste and errors: piloting lean principles at Intermountain Healthcare. Jt Comm J Qual Patient Saf 2005;31:249–57.
18. Kim CS, Spahlinger DA, Kin JM, et al. Lean health care: what can hospitals learn from a world-class automaker? J Hosp Med 2006;1:191–9.
19. Chalice R, American Society for Quality. Improving healthcare using Toyota lean production methods: 46 steps for improvement. 2nd edition. Milwaukee (WI): ASQ Quality Press; 2007.
20. Liker JK. The Toyota way: 14 management principles from the world's greatest manufacturer. New York: McGraw-Hill; 2004.
21. Liker JK, Meier D. The Toyota way fieldbook: a practical guide for implementing Toyota's 4Ps. New York: McGraw-Hill; 2006.
22. Reason JT. Human error. Cambridge (United Kingdom); New York: Cambridge University Press; 1990.
23. Milch CE, Salem DN, Pauker SG, et al. Voluntary electronic reporting of medical errors and adverse events. An analysis of 92,547 reports from 26 acute care hospitals. J Gen Intern Med 2006;21:165–70.
24. Wilmer A, Louie K, Dodek P, et al. Incidence of medication errors and adverse drug events in the ICU: a systematic review. Qual Saf Health Care 2010;19(5):e7.
25. Scanlon MC, Mistry KP, Jeffries HE. Determining pediatric intensive care unit quality indicators for measuring pediatric intensive care unit safety. Pediatr Crit Care Med 2007;8:S3–10.
26. Taylor JA, Brownstein D, Christakis DA, et al. Use of incident reports by physicians and nurses to document medical errors in pediatric patients. Pediatrics 2004;114:729–35.

27. Savage I, Cornford T, Klecun E, et al. Medication errors with electronic prescribing (eP): Two views of the same picture. BMC Health Serv Res 2010;10:135.
28. Reason J. Human error: models and management. BMJ 2000;320:768–70.
29. Resar RK, Rozich JD, Classen D. Methodology and rationale for the measurement of harm with trigger tools. Qual Saf Health Care 2003;12(Suppl 2):ii39–45.
30. Patient Safety Indicators Overview: AHRQ Quality Indicators. 2006. Available at: www.qualityindicators.ahrq.gov/psi_overview.htm. Accessed September 1, 2010.
31. McDonald KM, Davies SM, Haberland CA, et al. Preliminary assessment of pediatric health care quality and patient safety in the United States using readily available administrative data. Pediatrics 2008;122:e416–25.
32. Resar RK, Rozich JD, Simmonds T, et al. A trigger tool to identify adverse events in the intensive care unit. Jt Comm J Qual Patient Saf 2006;32:585–90.
33. Brilli RJ, McClead RE Jr, Davis T, et al. The Preventable Harm Index: an effective motivator to facilitate the drive to zero. J Pediatr 2010;157:681–3.
34. Winters B, Dorman T. Patient-safety and quality initiatives in the intensive-care unit. Curr Opin Anaesthesiol 2006;19:140–5.
35. Sandora TJ. Prevention of healthcare-associated infections in children: new strategies and success stories. Curr Opin Infect Dis 2010;23:300–5.
36. Miller MR, Griswold M, Harris JM 2nd, et al. Decreasing PICU catheter-associated bloodstream infections: NACHRI's quality transformation efforts. Pediatrics 2010;125:206–13.
37. A brief look at the new look at complex system failure, error, safety, and resilience. 2005. Available at: www.ctlab.org/documents/BriefLookAtTheNewLookVerAA.doc.pdf. Accessed September 1, 2010.
38. Pawson R, Tilley N. Realistic evaluation. London; Thousand Oaks (CA): Sage; 1997.
39. Godfrey MM, Melin CN, Muething SE, et al. Clinical microsystems, Part 3. Transformation of two hospitals using microsystem, mesosystem, and macrosystem strategies. Jt Comm J Qual Patient Saf 2008;34:591–603.
40. Shapiro S. Is meta-analysis a valid approach to the evaluation of small effects in observational studies? J Clin Epidemiol 1997;50:223–9.
41. Feinstein AR. Meta-analysis: statistical alchemy for the 21st century. J Clin Epidemiol 1995;48:71–9.
42. Bailar JC 3rd. The promise and problems of meta-analysis. N Engl J Med 1997; 337:559–61.
43. Huang DT, Clermont G, Kong L, et al. Intensive care unit safety culture and outcomes: a US multicenter study. Int J Qual Health Care 2010;22:151–61.
44. Pronovost PJ, Berenholtz SM, Goeschel C, et al. Improving patient safety in intensive care units in Michigan. J Crit Care 2008;23:207–21.
45. Pronovost P, Sexton B. Assessing safety culture: guidelines and recommendations. Qual Saf Health Care 2005;14:231–3.
46. Mohr DC, Burgess JF Jr, Young GJ. The influence of teamwork culture on physician and nurse resignation rates in hospitals. Health Serv Manage Res 2008;21: 23–31.
47. Jain M, Miller L, Belt D, et al. Decline in ICU adverse events, nosocomial infections and cost through a quality improvement initiative focusing on teamwork and culture change. Qual Saf Health Care 2006;15:235–9.
48. Abstoss K, Shaw B, Owens T, et al. Increasing medication error reporting rates while reducing harm through simultaneous cultural and system-level interventions in an intensive care unit. BMJ Qual Saf 2011;20:914–22.

49. Davidoff F. Heterogeneity is not always noise: lessons from improvement. JAMA 2009;302:2580–6.

50. Solberg LI, Mosser G, McDonald S. The three faces of performance measurement: improvement, accountability, and research. Jt Comm J Qual Improv 1997;23:135–47.

51. Berwick DM, Nolan TW. Physicians as leaders in improving health care: a new series in Annals of Internal Medicine. Ann Intern Med 1998;128:289–92.

52. Langley GJ. The improvement guide: a practical approach to enhancing organizational performance. 2nd edition. San Francisco: Jossey-Bass; 2009.

53. The Breakthrough Series: IHI's Collaborative Model for Achieving Breakthrough Improvement. IHI Innovation Series white paper. Boston; 2003. Available at: http://www.ihi.org/resources/pages/ihiwhitepapers/thebreakthroughseriesihiscollaborative modelforachievingbreakthroughimprovement.aspx. Accessed February 19, 2016.

54. Speroff T, O'Connor GT. Study designs for PDSA quality improvement research. Qual Manag Health Care 2004;13:17–32.

55. Benneyan JC, Lloyd RC, Plsek PE. Statistical process control as a tool for research and healthcare improvement. Qual Saf Health Care 2003;12: 458–64.

56. Mohammed MA, Worthington P, Woodall WH. Plotting basic control charts: tutorial notes for healthcare practitioners. Qual Saf Health Care 2008;17: 137–45.

57. Thor J, Lundberg J, Ask J, et al. Application of statistical process control in healthcare improvement: systematic review. Qual Saf Health Care 2007;16: 387–99.

58. Brilli RJ, Sparling KW, Lake MR, et al. The business case for preventing ventilator-associated pneumonia in pediatric intensive care unit patients. Jt Comm J Qual Patient Saf 2008;34:629–38.

59. Fox P, Porter PG, Lob SH, et al. Improving asthma-related health outcomes among low-income, multiethnic, school-aged children: results of a demonstration project that combined continuous quality improvement and community health worker strategies. Pediatrics 2007;120:e902–11.

60. Brilli RJ, Gibson R, Luria JW, et al. Implementation of a medical emergency team in a large pediatric teaching hospital prevents respiratory and cardiopulmonary arrests outside the intensive care unit. Pediatr Crit Care Med 2007;8:236–46 [quiz: 47].

61. Fu LY, Weissman M, McLaren R, et al. Improving the quality of immunization delivery to an at-risk population: a comprehensive approach. Pediatrics 2012; 129:e496–503.

62. Linam WM, Margolis PA, Atherton H, et al. Quality-improvement initiative sustains improvement in pediatric health care worker hand hygiene. Pediatrics 2011;128: e689–98.

63. Paul R, Melendez E, Stack A, et al. Improving adherence to PALS septic shock guidelines. Pediatrics 2014;133:e1358–66.

64. Marshall BC, Nelson EC. Accelerating implementation of biomedical research advances: critical elements of a successful 10 year Cystic Fibrosis Foundation healthcare delivery improvement initiative. BMJ Qual Saf 2014;23(Suppl 1): i95–103.

65. How-to guide: sustainability and spread. Cambridge (MA): Institute for Healthcare Improvement; 2011. Available at: http://www.ihi.org/resources/pages/ihiwhitepapers/thebreakthroughseriesihiscollaborativemodelforachievingbreak throughimprovement.aspx. Accessed February 19, 2016.

66. Improvement leader's guide to sustainability and spread. Cambridge (MA): Institute for Healthcare Improvement; 2011. Available at: http://www.ihi.org/resources/pages/ihiwhitepapers/fHowtoGuideSustainabilitySpread.aspx. Accessed February 19, 2016.
67. Levy FH, Brilli RJ, First LR, et al. A new framework for quality partnerships in children's hospitals. Pediatrics 2011;127:1147–56.
68. Billett AL, Colletti RB, Mandel KE, et al. Exemplar pediatric collaborative improvement networks: achieving results. Pediatrics 2013;131(Suppl 4):S196–203.

Big Data and Predictive Analytics
Applications in the Care of Children

Srinivasan Suresh, MD, MBA

KEYWORDS

- Big data • Predictive analytics • Clinical Informatics • Electronic Health Records

KEY POINTS

- Emerging changes in the United States' healthcare delivery model have led to renewed interest in data-driven methods for managing quality of care.
- Analytics (Data plus Information) plays a key role in predictive risk assessment, clinical decision support, and various patient throughput measures.
- The formation of clinical informatics as a formal board certified medical subspecialty is a key step towards the development of physician informaticists who can leverage information technology to improve the delivery and safety of healthcare.
- The combination of big data and predictive analytics in healthcare has the great potential to positively affect clinical decision support, patient morbidity, and hospital operations such as cost management systems and resource allocation.

"Big data" is a broad term for collection of data sets so large and complex that they are difficult to process using on-hand database management tools or traditional data processing applications.[1] Predictive analytics encompasses a variety of statistical techniques from modeling, machine learning, and data mining that analyze current and historical facts to make predictions about the future, or otherwise unknown events.[2]

Changes in the health care delivery model over the past decade in the United States have led to renewed interest and newer mechanisms in data-driven methods for managing quality of care. Health systems and provider groups are now evaluated using quality metrics for mortality, length of stay, and for hospital readmissions within 30 days. Rankings are increasingly made public, and are being used by insurers to institute pay-for-performance programs.[3] Hospitals need to continually monitor and understand their performance, and determine whether interventions to improve have been successful.

Disclosures: None.
Children's Hospital of Pittsburgh, 4401 Penn Avenue, Room 6415 AOB, Pittsburgh, PA 15224, USA
E-mail address: suresh@chp.edu

Pediatr Clin N Am 63 (2016) 357–366
http://dx.doi.org/10.1016/j.pcl.2015.12.007
0031-3955/16/$ – see front matter © 2016 Elsevier Inc. All rights reserved.

DEFINITION OF ANALYTICS AND ITS IMPACT ON HEALTH CARE

Analytics is the systematic use of data combined with quantitative as well as qualitative analysis to make decisions. Health care analytics efficiently applies clinical and administrative data in electronic health records (EHRs), and knowledge of clinical practice standards and guidelines, by way of order sets and protocols, to manage metric-driven quality improvement. The goals of such an initiative are to identify inefficiencies in care delivery and variations from standard practice, explore opportunities for expanding services that may enhance quality of care, efficient targeting of limited resources, and peer benchmarking. The analytical techniques needed to achieve these goals require mature EHR implementations.[4]

EHRs with the required breadth of data increasingly are available at children's hospitals. Institutions may make these data available through a clinical data warehouse, a relational database fed by an EHR's transactional system that supports efficient population queries. National repositories of administrative and sometimes clinical data provide institutions with access to comparative data; for example, the Children's Hospital Association (CHA) Pediatric Health Information System (PHIS). The CHA, through a wide variety of data programs, helps pediatric hospitals drive improved clinical, operational, and financial performance. With shared data sets, potentially better practices across organizations can be identified, ultimately improving children's health care. The PHIS, a comparative pediatric database, includes clinical and resource use data for inpatient, ambulatory surgery, emergency department, and observation unit patient encounters for 45 children's hospitals.[5] PHIS supports a wide range of improvement activities, including clinical effectiveness, resource use, care guideline development, readmission analysis, antimicrobial stewardship, and physician profiling (ongoing professional practice evaluation). Such data sets represent a rich potential source of data for analytics, but they also present substantial challenges in their use. Diagnoses, comorbidities, and procedures typically are represented indirectly as billing codes.[6] Clinical data such as laboratory test results and medication histories may be recorded as local codes or in text, and they may require substantial clinical context to interpret. Efforts are underway to create publicly available libraries of phenotypes defined in terms of patterns in codes and discrete data.[7] Tools for translating these phenotypes into queries of local data warehouses and national repositories could make data-driven quality improvement more broadly practical.

ANALYTICS IN THE FORM OF DECISION SUPPORT AND MONITORING SYSTEMS

Analytics play a key role in predictive risk assessment, clinical decision support, home health monitoring, finance, and resource allocation.[8] They may also be used to enhance less sophisticated, rules-based systems that are already in use. One of the benefits of EHRs has been the integration of clinical decision support (CDS) systems. CDS systems have been shown to reduce errors and improve clinical outcomes in certain settings, such as pediatric intensive care units,[9] and can result in performance improvement on perioperative quality and process measures. Some CDS systems that are designed to prevent medication errors are based largely on commercially available software packages that rely on simple rules. Often, these products do not provide ideal rule sensitivity, and institutions must perform manual reclassification of drug-drug interactions to improve the efficacy of their CDS systems. Analytics may offer a solution to this challenge, because clinicians can use analytics techniques to query and mine the EHR for meaningful connections, and then synergistically combine the knowledge-based rules with analytics applied to EHR data.[10]

Analytics are used in health care applications outside of the traditional inpatient and outpatient care settings, such as wearable monitors that patients use at home. Wearable health monitoring systems consist of a variety of sensors, actuators, and multimedia devices, and enable low-cost, noninvasive options for continuous monitoring of health, activity, mobility, and mental status, both indoors and outdoors. Thus, wearable monitoring systems provide continuous physiologic data that may reflect the general health of the monitored individuals, and the use of wearable sensors in health monitoring systems is an emerging field that necessitates data mining and analytics of physiologic measurements in a nonclinical setting.[11] Such health monitoring systems may reduce health care costs by disease prevention and enhance the quality of life with disease management.

ARCHITECTURAL FRAMEWORK

The conceptual framework for a big data analytics project in health care is similar to that of a traditional health informatics or analytics project. The key difference lies in how processing is executed. In a regular health analytics project, the analysis can be performed with a business intelligence tool installed on a stand-alone system, such as a desktop or laptop. Because big data are by definition large, processing is broken down and executed across multiple nodes. The concept of distributed processing has existed for decades. What is new is its use in analyzing very large data sets as health care providers start to tap into their large data repositories to gain insight for making better-informed health-related decisions. In addition, open-source platforms such as Hadoop/MapReduce, available on the cloud, have encouraged the application of big data analytics in health care. By discovering associations and understanding patterns and trends within the data, big data analytics has the potential to improve care, save lives, and reduce costs.[12]

The volume and variety of health care–related data continue to grow, spurred on by the increasing adoption and use of EHRs, the expansion of omics data, and the proliferation of actigraphy data from wearable self-tracking devices and mobile applications. The use of these data for health care analytics such as data visualization, patient stratification, predictive modeling, personalized medicine, and drug discovery will increasingly depend on the ability to appropriately collect, curate, and integrate disparate data from many different sources. The linking of many different types of data will allow the analysis and modeling of complex multidimensional interactions that can enable deeper insights. A robust data collection, curation, and integration infrastructure should comprise the following stages: data collection, data understanding, data validation, data cleaning, data integration, and data enrichment.[13]

Beyond early detection of disease, predictive modeling can also facilitate greater individualization of care. Predictive models can enable clinicians to distinguish individuals who will benefit from a specific therapeutic intervention from those that will not. For example, it is known that obesity, with or without the metabolic syndrome, increases children's risk for developing diabetes, but most of these children do not develop diabetes. The ability to refine the predictive ability for developing diabetes would allow therapies to be better targeted to the individuals most likely to benefit. As the understanding of genomic information increases, the combination of genomic, environmental, and clinical variables in predictive modeling is likely to be critical for the individualization of care in a broad array of disease processes.[14]

DATA SCIENTISTS

The primary value of analytics to end users in health care is the access to actionable information, which needs to be synthesized from various data sources. A personnel resource that has come to the forefront lately is the data scientist, who is an expert analyst, and can serve as a 1-stop shop for data management, analysis, and interpretation of electronic data. In health care, this is particularly important for translating electronic bits into meaningful data. These data scientists need to be proficient in a broad spectrum of analytical methodologies that encompass traditional (biostatistics, epidemiology, discrete-event simulation, and causal modeling) as well as emerging methods (data mining, bayesian statistics, optimization modeling, social network analysis, and agent-based simulation).[15]

ANALYTICS IN HOSPITAL OPERATIONS

Analytics can play a vital role in hospitals' cost management systems, not only in cost savings based on improved patient care and outcomes but also in the identification of simple billing anomalies (ie, revenue leakage). Most health care organizations find billing anomalies via a combination of rules-based approaches and manual audits. However, this approach is time consuming and error prone. Advanced analytics approaches (eg, machine learning and predictive modeling) can be used to find patterns in billing records that are most likely associated with missing or erroneous charges.[16]

In other data-driven revolutions, some players have taken advantage of data transparency by pursuing objectives that create value only for themselves. In health care, some stakeholders may try to take advantage of big data more quickly and aggressively than their competitors, without regard to clinically proven outcomes. Such risks are real and possibly unavoidable. As such, patients, providers, and payors pursuing the appropriate influence levers will be wise to be alert for such abuses and demand to see the related evidence showing that certain services are essential.[17]

ADVANCED ANALYTICS/CLINICAL DECISION SUPPORT

At Children's Hospital of Pittsburgh of the University of Pittsburgh Medical Center (UPMC), an analytical tool that is used as an early warning sign for clinical deterioration is the Pediatric Rothman Index (pRI). The software uses existing data in the patient's electronic medical record (EMR), in conjunction with a live data feed from patients' continuous monitoring systems, and generates a graph displaying patient's condition based on laboratory results; vital signs; and, more importantly, nursing assessments. The trends update every 1, 5, and 60 minutes based on the unit requirements.

The Rothman Index graphs can draw attention to gradual but important health declines that can be difficult to detect when a patient is handed off between multiple physicians and nurses. In addition, by providing an objective number, it is possible to more effectively deploy rapid response teams. This measurement (on a scale of 0–100) is a visual alert that brings attention to patients who are categorized as very high risk, high risk, and medium risk. These alerts provide multiple opportunities to potentially pick up critical conditions up to 12 hours before they are observed by conventional assessments.

The pRI is a universal patient score, identifying a patient's condition in real time, with an easy-to-understand composite score. The key features are that it is (1) universal, so it can be used across most disease categories and patient populations. (2) Simple; pRI is a number from 0 to 100, and can be trended easily. (3) Automated; calculated using existing data from the EMR. (4) Real time; automatically calculated from EMR data, and reported in real time. (5) Integrated with the hospital's EMR. **Fig. 1** shows the time frame between the electronic alert (firing of the index, which can be set at predefined levels) and clinical deterioration as defined by conventional means.

Dashboards that distill and convey vast amounts of data in a format that is valuable to clinical and administrative leaders are an important analytical tool. These self-service tools can provide clinical, demographic, throughput, quality-of-care, and financial metrics on demand, thereby enabling peer benchmarking, both at the individual physician level and at the interhospital level. This ability can lead to standardizing care, reducing unnecessary variation, and potentially limiting costs of care. Such models typically overlay electronic record systems, patient registration systems, and cost management systems and extract structured data. **Fig. 2** shows an example of an advanced dashboard for a specific disease management system (appendicitis), and **Fig. 3** shows an early version of a population health module.

Another area in hospital operations that disproportionately consumes resources is readmissions. Although the impact to the financial bottom line may not as heavy as in primarily adult hospitals, readmissions in children's hospitals are starting to face claims denials, and place a burden to the provider, the patient, and health care as a whole. At Children's Hospital of Pittsburgh of UPMC, we are developing readmission prediction models that are built on machine learning techniques. These models are expected to target common pediatric illnesses that are also leading causes of readmissions, such as seizure disorder, acute asthma exacerbation, and pneumonia. The algorithms that predict the probability of readmissions take into account numerous variables from every admission and provide the risk number in the patient's electronic record in a dynamic fashion, at point of care. This process allows discharging physicians to plan postdischarge care coordination (which could include the follow-up visit with the primary care physician or with a subspecialist, or care on subsequent days at home by a visiting nurse). This application specifically highlights the power of big data and predictive analytics combined. **Fig. 4** shows a screenshot of the readmission prediction application in the physician view of the EMR.

GENOMICS AND BIG DATA

Advances in genomics such as high-throughput sequencing technology are causing a significant reduction in the cost and effort of sequencing the human genome

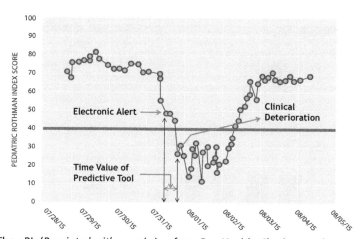

Fig. 1. The pRI. (*Reprinted with* permission from PeraHealth, Charlotte NC).

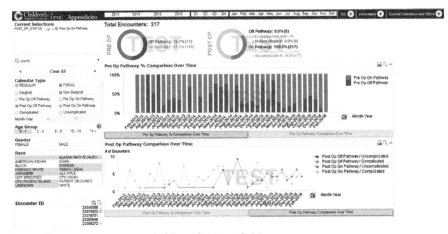

Fig. 2. Disease management dashboard: appendicitis.

(encompassing 30,000–35,000 genes).[18] With implications for current public health policies and delivery of care, analyzing genome-scale data for developing actionable recommendations in a timely manner is a significant challenge to computational biology. Cost and time to deliver recommendations are crucial in a clinical setting. Initiatives tackling this complex problem include tracking of 100,000 subjects over 20 to 30 years using the predictive, preventive, participatory, and personalized health, referred to as P4, medicine paradigm[19] as well as an integrative personal omics profile.[20] The P4 initiative is using a system approach for (1) analyzing genome-scale data sets to determine disease states; (2) moving toward blood-based diagnostic tools for continuous monitoring of patients; (3) exploring new approaches to drug target discovery, developing tools to deal with big data challenges of capturing, validating, storing, mining, and integrating data; and then (4) modeling data for each individual. The integrative personal omics profile combines physiologic monitoring and multiple high-throughput methods for genome sequencing to generate detailed health and disease states for patients. Using such high-density data for exploration, discovery, and clinical translation demands novel big data approaches and analytics.[21]

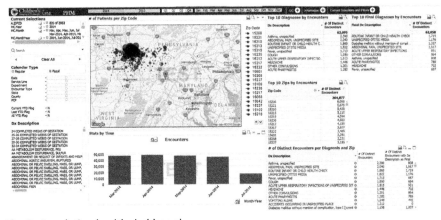

Fig. 3. Population health dashboard.

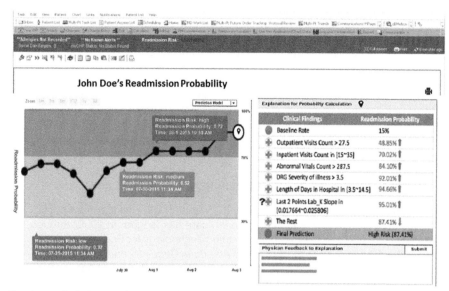

Fig. 4. Readmission prediction application (embedded in the EMR at the patient level).

The resources needed for data collection and secure maintenance could be daunting for most hospitals. A critical rate-limiting factor in the application of large data sets is the quality of the collected data, because the consequences of analyzing erroneous data cannot be mitigated even by advanced statistical techniques.[22]

THE PERSONALIZED MEDICINE COALITION

The concept of personalized medicine (that medical care can be tailored to the genomic and molecular profile of the individual) has repercussions that extend far beyond the technology that makes it possible. The adoption of personalized medicine will require changes in health care infrastructure, diagnostics and therapeutics business models, reimbursement policy from government and private payors, and a different approach to regulatory oversight. Personalized medicine will shift medical practices upstream from the reactive treatment of disease to proactive health care management, including screening, early treatment, and prevention, and will alter the roles of both physician and patient. It will create a greater reliance on EMRs and decision support systems in an industry that has a long history of resistance to information technology.

Personalized medicine requires a systems approach to implementation. However, in a health care economy that is highly decentralized and market driven, it is incumbent on the stakeholders to advocate for a consistent set of policies and legislation that pave the way for the adoption of personalized medicine. To address this need, the Personalized Medicine Coalition (PMC) was formed as a nonprofit umbrella organization of pharmaceutical, biotechnology, diagnostic, and information technology companies; health care providers and payors; patient advocacy groups; industry policy organizations; major academic institutions; and government agencies. The PMC provides a structure for achieving consensus positions among these stakeholders on crucial public policy issues; a role that will be vital to translating personalized medicine into widespread clinical practice.[23]

IMPACT ON DIAGNOSTIC IMAGING

A strategic plan for big data in medical imaging is to dynamically integrate medical images, in vitro diagnostic information, genetic information, EHRs, and clinical notes into patients' profiles. This integration provides the ability for personalized decision support by the analysis of data from large numbers of patients with similar conditions. A medical report can be built with context-specific and target group–specific information that requires access and analysis of big data. The report can be created with the help of semantic technology, which is an umbrella term used to describe natural language processing, data mining, artificial intelligence, tagging, and searching by concept instead of by key word.[24]

CHALLENGES AND FUTURE OF ANALYTICS IN HEALTH CARE

Despite the role of information technology (IT) in rapidly advancing the productivity of other service industries, IT adoption in health care has lagged. In 2009, through the Affordable Care Act, and the Health Information Technology for Economic and Clinical Health Act, which was a component of the American Recovery and Reinvestment Act, the US government set aside a sizable investment in health IT that has incentivized eligible hospitals and providers to meet meaningful-use regulations in order to improve the quality of care.[25] This investment has resulted in a perceptible increase in the collection of patient data in electronic form. The next phase is to transform these data into actionable information packets that can be used to improve the delivery of health care.

There are numerous challenges to the application and use of analytics; namely, the lack of data standards, barriers to the collection of high-quality data, and a shortage of qualified personnel to conduct such analyses. There are also multiple managerial issues, such as how to get end users of electronic data to use it consistently for improving health care delivery, and how to manage the public reporting and sharing of data.

A challenge presented by data is not only quantitative (ie, managing massive data files) but also qualitative. For example, terabytes of data can be generated in rapid fashion by a hospital floor full of electronic patient monitors; however, each type of physiologic monitor (eg, pulse oximetry, capnography) is subject to artifact. The subsequent application of analytics to data artifacts may produce faulty conclusions (ie, garbage in, garbage out). One potential solution to this problem is the application of analytics, such as machine learning and neural networks, in data auditing to detect errors before analysis.

Discussions of big data in medicine often revolve around gene sequencing and biosamples. It is perhaps less recognized that administrative data in the form of vital records, hospital discharge abstracts, insurance claims, and other routinely collected data also offer the potential for using information from hundreds of thousands, if not millions, of people to answer important questions. However, the increasing ease with which such data may be used and reused has increased concerns about privacy and informed consent. Addressing these concerns without creating insurmountable barriers to the use of such data for research is essential in pediatrics data science.[26]

THE SPECIALTY OF CLINICAL INFORMATICS AND BOARD CERTIFICATION

The proliferation of EHRs has resulted in massive amounts of data for hospitals and health care organizations to manage and analyze for various purposes, including practice management, quality improvement, and outcomes research projects, which has led to increased demand for professionals who are well versed in both informatics and medicine. To meet this demand, the American Medical Informatics Association spearheaded the establishment of professional-level education and certification for physicians in informatics, leading to development of clinical informatics as a formal, board-certified medical subspecialty.[27]

Clinical informatics professionals leverage IT to improve the delivery and safety of health care via EHRs, telemedicine, and evidence-based medicine using tools such as CDSs and data analytics. Patient-generated health data provide a promising approach to personalized health care, as well as medical diagnostics, via data mining and the development of computer-aided diagnostic tools. The future of health care analytics will consist of an ever-increasing demand for application of sophisticated analytics methods and tools (eg, visual analytics dashboards) to explore and analyze data with the goals of improving patient care, increasing efficiency, optimizing resource use and allocation, and enhancing decision making at both the clinical and enterprise levels. Health care professionals with knowledge and expertise in clinical informatics will be needed to design and implement the future analytical applications and innovations of EHR and communication systems to meet those needs.

IMPACT ON QUALITY OF LIFE

In conclusion, the combination of big data and predictive analytics can lead to treatments that specifically work for individual children, provide the ability to prescribe medications that work for each individual, and are not given unnecessarily just because that medication works for most people. The patient's role will change as patients become more informed consumers who work with their physicians collaboratively to achieve better outcomes. Patients could become aware of possible personal health risks sooner because of alerts from their genome analysis, from predictive models relayed by their physicians, from the increasing use of apps and wearables, and because of better accuracy in the information that is needed for accurate predictions. This awareness will empower them to make lifestyle changes, positively affecting their future well-being.[28]

REFERENCES

1. Available at: https://en.wikipedia.org/wiki/Big_data. Accessed February 20, 2016.
2. Available at: https://en.wikipedia.org/wiki/Predictive_analytics. Accessed February 20, 2016.
3. Lindenauer PK, Remus D, Roman S, et al. Public reporting and pay for performance in hospital quality improvement. N Engl J Med 2007;356:486–96.
4. Post AR, Kurc T, Cholleti S, et al. The analytic information warehouse: a platform for analytics using electronic health record data. J Biomed Inform 2013;46(3): 410–24.
5. Children's Hospital Association. Pediatric health information system. Available at: https://www.childrenshospitals.org/Programs-and-Services/Data-Analytics-and-Research/Pediatric-Health-Information-System. Accessed February 20, 2016.
6. O'Malley KJ, Cook KF, Price MD, et al. Measuring diagnoses: ICD code accuracy. Health Serv Res 2005;40:1620–39.
7. Pathak J, Wang J, Kashyap S, et al. Mapping clinical phenotype data elements to standardized metadata repositories and controlled terminologies: the eMERGE Network experience. J Am Med Inform Assoc 2011;18:376–86.
8. Simpao AF, Ahumada LM, Gálvez JA, et al. A review of analytics and clinical informatics in health care. J Med Syst 2014;38:45.

9. van Rosse F, Maat B, Rademaker CM, et al. The effect of computerized physician order entry on medication prescription errors and clinical outcome in pediatric and intensive care: a systematic review. Pediatrics 2009;123:1184–90.

10. Slonimc N, Carmeli B, Goldsteen A, et al. Knowledge-analytics synergy in clinical decision support. Stud Health Technol Inform 2012;180:703–7.

11. Banaee H, Ahmed MU, Loutfi A. Data mining for wearable sensors in health monitoring systems: a review of recent trends and challenges. Sensors 2013;13:17472–500.

12. Raghupathi W, Raghupathi V. Big data analytics in healthcare: promise and potential. Health Inf Sci Syst 2014;2:3. Available at: http://www.hissjournal.com/content/2/1/3.

13. Ng K, Kakkanatt C, Benigno M, et al. Curating and integrating data from multiple sources to support healthcare analytics. Stud Health Technol Inform 2015;216:1056.

14. Ng K, Ghoting A, Steinhubl SR, et al. PARAMO: a parallel predictive modeling platform for healthcare analytic research using electronic health records. J Biomed Inform 2014;48:160–70.

15. Ward MJ, Marsolo KA, Froehle CM. Applications of business analytics in healthcare. Bus Horiz 2014;57(5):571–82.

16. Schouten P. Big data in health care: solving provider revenue leakage with advanced analytics. Healthc Financ Manage 2013;67:40–2.

17. Groves P, Kayyali B, Knott D, Van Kuiken S. The 'big data' revolution in healthcare. McKinsey & Company. Center for US Health System Reform, Business Technology Office; 2013.

18. Drmanac R, Sparks AB, Callow MJ, et al. Human genome sequencing using unchained base reads on self-assembling DNA nanoarrays. Science 2010;327(5961):78–81.

19. Hood L, Friend SH. Predictive, personalized, preventive, participatory (P4) cancer medicine. Nat Rev Clin Oncol 2011;8(3):184–7.

20. Chen R, Mias GI, Li-Pook-Than J, et al. Personal omics profiling reveals dynamic molecular and medical phenotypes. Cell 2012;148(6):1293–307.

21. Belle A, Thiagarajan R, Soroushmehr SM, et al. Big data analytics in healthcare. Biomed Res Int 2015;2015:370194.

22. Janke AT, Overbeek DL, Kocher KE, et al. Exploring the potential of predictive analytics and big data in emergency care. Ann Emerg Med 2016;67(2):227–36.

23. Abrahams E, Ginsburg GS, Silver M. The personalized medicine coalition: goals and strategies. Am J Pharmacogenomics 2005;5(6):345–55.

24. Available at: http://www.diagnosticimaging.com/siim-2014/big-data-expected-have-big-impact-diagnostic-imaging. Accessed February 20, 2016.

25. Stark P. Congressional intent for the HITECH Act. Am J Manag Care 2010;16:24–8.

26. Currie J. Big data versus big brother: on the appropriate use of large-scale data collections in pediatrics. Pediatrics 2013;131:S127.

27. Lehmann CU, Shorte V, Gundlapalli AV. Clinical informatics sub-specialty board certification. Pediatr Rev 2013;34:525–30.

28. Winters-Miner LA. Seven ways predictive analytics can improve healthcare. Available at: https://www.elsevier.com/connect/seven-ways-predictive-analytics-can-improve-healthcare. Accessed February 20, 2016.

Pediatric Telehealth
Opportunities and Challenges

Levon Utidjian, MD, MBI[a,b,*], Erika Abramson, MD, MS[c,d]

KEYWORDS

- Telehealth • Telemedicine • Pediatrics • Access to care • mHealth

KEY POINTS

- Telehealth is a rapidly expanding field of medicine that uses telecommunication and information technology to connect patients and providers remotely.
- Telehealth has significant potential to improve population health by expanding access to care, improving communication, facilitating enhanced monitoring of patients, and expanding educational opportunities.
- To continue to capitalize on the benefits of telehealth, barriers including lack of infrastructure, licensing issues, security and privacy issues, and legal concerns must be addressed.

INTRODUCTION

Telehealth is a rapidly growing field of medicine that uses telecommunication and information technology to assist in the delivery of health care to patients at a distance from providers. These technologies can help connect patients with providers, and providers with other providers, such as subspecialists, to improve patient access to care and provider access to subspecialist expertise and knowledge sources. As telecommunications and computer technology have become increasingly reliable and inexpensive, the methods of communication have expanded beyond just telephone calls between patient and provider to include videoconferencing, the exchange of high-resolution image and video files, and the ability to remotely monitor patients via the Internet.

Disclosure Statement: The authors have identified no professional or financial affiliations for themselves or their spouse/partner.

[a] Department of Pediatrics, The Children's Hospital of Philadelphia, Perelman School of Medicine at the University of Pennsylvania, 34th Street & Civic Center Boulevard, Philadelphia, PA 19104, USA; [b] Department of Biomedical and Health Informatics, The Children's Hospital of Philadelphia, 3535 Market Street, Suite 1024, Room 1080, Philadelphia, PA 19104, USA; [c] Department of Pediatrics, Weill Cornell Medicine, 525 E 68th Street, Rm M610A, New York, NY 10065, USA; [d] Healthcare Policy and Research, Weill Cornell Medicine, 402 East 67th Street, New York, NY, 10065, USA

* Corresponding author. Department of Biomedical and Health Informatics, The Children's Hospital of Philadelphia, 3535 Market Street, Suite 1024, Room 1080, Philadelphia, PA 19104.

E-mail address: utidjianl@email.chop.edu

Pediatr Clin N Am 63 (2016) 367–378
http://dx.doi.org/10.1016/j.pcl.2015.11.006
0031-3955/16/$ – see front matter

pediatric.theclinics.com

In the last decade, governmental and public support for the use of telehealth technology has continued to increase. In 2010, the Patient Protection and Affordable Care Act (ACA) included provisions that promoted the use of telehealth by Accountable Care Organizations, and in the care of behavioral health issues and patients with chronic, complex conditions.[1] As of 2012, approximately 10 million patients were receiving telehealth services annually in the United States.[2] Although that is a small percentage of the total US population, the number is expected to only increase. For example, a recent 2015 survey showed that 64% of patients were willing to have a remote medical video visit.[3] Another factor likely to stimulate interest in telehealth services is the acceptance of these offerings by large US employers: in 2014, only 48% offered telehealth services to employees, but by 2016 the percentage of participating companies is expected to rise to 74%.[4]

Pediatric medicine is expected to benefit from the use of telehealth technology by improving patient access to care in underserved rural areas, and extending the reach of pediatric subspecialists at academic and tertiary medical centers to patients and colleagues in more distant community hospitals and clinics. A recent American Academy of Pediatrics (AAP) policy statement on the expanding role of telehealth in pediatrics highlights the ability of this technology to improve aspects of pediatric care and help deal with workforce shortages.[5] This article explores how telehealth can be used to improve pediatric health care quality and safety. It also examines the current challenges to the successful implementation of telehealth that must still be overcome to help the field reach its full potential.

DEFINING TELEHEALTH

To define telehealth, one must first begin with the term telemedicine, which has been in use since the 1960s. Although telecommunication systems, such as the telegraph, radio, and telephone, were coming in to use by medical providers well before then, the use of systems to transmit patient data, such as telemetry-based vital sign monitoring, really began to emerge during the manned-space flight program.[6] As the novel uses of telecommunications and other types of information exchange continued to multiply in medicine, the Institute of Medicine came to define telemedicine as "the use of electronic information and communications technologies to provide and support healthcare when distance separates the participants."[7] Although "distance" is traditionally viewed in terms of geography, such as between a remote rural area and an urban medical center, telemedicine may also be used across shorter distances, even within the same town or city, when time or convenience is an issue.

Although telemedicine usually refers to the delivery of direct patient care services, the term telehealth encompasses a wider range of services, including the clinical services of telemedicine in addition to nonclinical ones.[8] Examples of such nonclinical uses include provider training and continuing education, and administrative purposes. Despite these distinctions, the terms telemedicine and telehealth are often viewed as synonymous and used interchangeably.[9] As such, for the rest of this article, the term telehealth is used. Additional useful resources for information about telehealth organizations and information are provided in **Box 1**.

CLASSIFYING TELEHEALTH SERVICES

Telehealth services come in many different forms, but can usually be divided into one of two types based on the timing of the interaction.[10] Asynchronous services do not involve real-time interaction, but rather the storage and forwarding of clinical data between participants. Examples of such services are teledermatology and

---

Box 1
Useful resources

- American Telemedicine Association
  - http://www.americantelemed.org
  - A leading international advocate and resource promoting telehealth
- Telehealth Resource Center
  - http://www.telehealthresourcecenter.org
  - Provide assistance and education and information to organizations and individuals who are actively providing or interested in engaging in telehealth
- Health Resources and Services Administration Telehealth
  - http://www.hrsa.gov/ruralhealth/telehealth/
  - Resource page on telehealth, including information about grant opportunities
- Agency for Health Information Technology Telehealth
  - https://healthit.ahrq.gov/key-topics/telehealth
  - Includes background information and descriptions of current Agency-funded projects related to telehealth

---

teleradiology wherein images are sent to dermatologists and radiologists, respectively, who then review the images and respond with a diagnostic interpretation on their own time.[2] These asynchronous services can also involve other media, such as audio and video recordings. This is in contrast to synchronous services that require real-time interaction between participants, such as teleconsultation using videoconferencing technology between a provider and patient, or a provider and subspecialist. Relevant patient information may also be sent during such synchronous interactions, but the discussion of the patient happens in real-time to allow immediate feedback and follow-up questions.

Common types of telehealth services can also be distinguished by participant location. Home-based services involve patients at home or a nursing care facility that require the remote monitoring of physiologic data or test results, such as blood sugars.[2,11] Office- or hospital-based services include virtual medical visits between the patient and provider by videoconference or a provider pursuing teleconsultation with a specialist.[11] Participants can also access services beyond the confines of a specific location with cell phones, tablet computers, and other mobile technology being used as mobile health (mHealth) devices. Some mHealth applications include remote medical consultation, reminders to improve medication compliance, and communication of other educational materials in the field, outside the home and office.[12]

OPPORTUNITIES TO IMPROVE QUALITY OF CARE AND PATIENT SAFETY

Telehealth has the potential to improve the quality of care and patient safety in pediatrics. These include ways to improve patient access to care, extend provider outreach, increase education for all participants, and reduce resource use throughout the health care system. These opportunities are summarized in **Table 1**.

Patient Access to Care

One of the most immediate expected benefits of telehealth is the ability to increase patient access to care by delivering it when and where patients need it. The AAP policy statement notes that there exists a significant disparity in the distribution of pediatricians and subspecialists across the United States, leading to underserved regions.[5] Apart from overcoming geographic barriers, parents are also likely to consider

Table 1
Potential benefits of telehealth technology

Aspects of Care	Potential Benefits
Patient access to care	• Telehealth can help improve access in underserved regions • Better accommodation of parent work schedules • Strengthening the medical home
Provider outreach	• Enhance rural provider relationships with subspecialists • Pediatric subspecialists at children's hospitals and tertiary centers can support and guide care in nonpediatric inpatient and emergency department settings
Patient, family, and provider education	• Patients and their families can receive additional training on chronic disease management • Providers can gain new patient management skills from subspecialists • Providers can participate in continuing medical education and other web-based learning activities
Resource utilization	• Cost savings from avoiding unnecessary transports between health care facilities • Avoiding redundant diagnostic testing • Reduction of unnecessary referrals by prescreening • Reduction of child school and parent work absences

telehealth options that could prove more convenient around their work schedules or be more time efficient. A recent survey asked what treatment options consumers would consider for middle-of-the-night care, and 30% of parents with children in the home would select a video visit compared with only 18% of adults without children.[3]

Pediatric care has been shown to be particularly amenable to telehealth services. A telehealth model demonstrated that approximately 85% of acute visits to ambulatory pediatric clinics could be managed as telehealth encounters, even if they required such procedures as simple in-office laboratory testing or albuterol treatments.[13] Subspecialty teleconsultations have proved to be effective for various types of encounters including autism evaluation, cardiology, dermatology, and retinopathy of prematurity screening.[14–18] Given the scarcity of many pediatric subspecialists, telehealth services might be a less expensive or time-consuming option for patients in remote underserved areas.

In addition to certain telehealth services proving to be as clinically effective as in-person encounters, patient satisfaction with such services is also reported to be high. A systematic review of patient satisfaction with telehealth services found that all 32 examined studies showed good levels of patient satisfaction.[19] Another benefit for patients is that such improved access to care can also help lead to better, safer care by supporting the patient-centered medical home (PCMH). By offering telehealth services, primary care providers can help avoid fragmentation of care by patients seeking services at standalone walk-in clinics or urgent care centers. Keeping care within the PCMH leads to a more complete medical record, better continuity of care, and closer follow-up by a patient's primary care provider.[20]

Provider Outreach

Just as patients are expected to benefit from increased access to care, telehealth technology enables providers to offer more services and higher quality care to their patients. Because only 5% of US hospitals are children's hospitals, most children receive care in nonpediatric specialized hospitals.[21] Telehealth services can help extend the expertise of pediatricians and subspecialists at children's hospitals and large tertiary care centers by enabling them to reach providers and community hospitals in remote settings. This can in turn empower those providers to care for their patients without having to refer them to other specialists or transfer them to other hospitals. Interviews conducted in 2013 with rural pediatricians showed that they were strongly supportive of multiple telehealth strategies, so long as the goal was to enhance rather than replace relationships between rural pediatricians and subspecialists.[22]

Several studies have examined how telehealth extends the abilities of providers in the delivery of care in intensive care unit (ICU) and emergency department (ED) settings to provide better, safer care. The use of remote-controlled, robotic telehealth technology for rounding in a neonatal ICU was shown to be effective at managing patients and could help provide complementary support to underserved neonatal ICUs.[23] Teleconsultations between pediatric critical care specialists and remote providers in adult ICUs caring for children led to similar severity-adjusted mortality rates, and improved adherence to pediatric critical care best practices and treatment guidelines.[24,25] Similar teleconsultations between pediatric critical care specialists and providers in nonpediatric EDs were also shown to be useful in dealing with seriously ill patients and, in one study, even improved patient safety by leading to fewer physician-related ED medication errors.[26,27]

Patient, Family, and Provider Education

Telehealth technology can also provide new ways to educate patients and their families on managing diseases themselves, and provide continuing medical education (CME) for providers. Streaming videos and interactive websites can be used to engage patients in learning about self-management of chronic conditions. The use of telehealth technology to provide patient education for such diseases as asthma and diabetes has led to increased patient knowledge of their disease and improvement in objective measures of clinical outcomes.[28] The use of mHealth text messaging programs to educate people about human immunodeficiency virus/AIDS in the developing world has resulted in increased disease awareness and rates of human immunodeficiency virus/AIDS testing.[12]

Providers can also benefit from educational offerings that can reach them in remote locations. Online educational sources can include academic lectures, clinical conferences, journal clubs, or other CME programs. Lectures can be delivered synchronously via videoconferencing and thus allow providers to have discussions with other colleagues. Such interactions with clinical content experts and subspecialists can help providers develop greater expertise to manage complex patients on their own, and promote networking among medical professionals. Storing such programs online would enable asynchronous delivery of these materials so that providers could use them at their own convenience and still benefit from them. Results from a pediatric medicine telehealth educational program in the state of Arkansas showed that online delivery of CME materials was well received by participants who believed the materials were relevant to their professional needs, increased their knowledge, and would influence their clinical practice.[29]

Resource Utilization

Since the passage of the ACA, there is greater pressure on the health care system to find new ways to provide high-quality care more efficiently. Telehealth services have the potential to meet that goal by reducing costs through better communication of patient information. Not only is information relatively inexpensive to transmit compared with the physical transport of patients, but telehealth also provides additional savings to patients, their families, and society apart from direct health care costs.

A direct financial benefit of telehealth's ability to overcome the distance between patients and providers is the avoidance of the costs of transporting patients between health care facilities. Given that the transportation of medically complex patients requiring life support and close monitoring is expensive and not without risk, a telehealth service that could extend the reach of experts at lower cost and without endangering patients would seem to provide cost savings and more efficient care delivery. A pediatric ICU telehealth program providing pediatric critical care expertise to rural adult ICUs demonstrated an ability of such an intervention to keep more patients in house and avoid unnecessary transports.[30] This resulted in large cost savings from the difference in ICU costs between hospitals and avoided transport costs, which accounted for two-thirds of the annual savings of the telehealth program.

Telehealth services can also lead to better use of limited resources, such as the availability of subspecialist appointments, by providing a more efficient way to communicate between providers. Telehealth programs that offer a means for providers to discuss patient cases with subspecialists have been shown to provide many benefits and cost-savings.[31,32] The ability to obtain specialist input on a patient can lead to early initiation of diagnostic testing and treatments by the primary care provider while the patient waits to be seen by the subspecialist, increasing the efficiency of care delivery. This can also lead to avoidance of unnecessary and redundant diagnostic procedures if the subspecialist can direct the work-up at a distance. An unexpected benefit of such telehealth programs is that it can actually avoid the need for the patient to even visit the subspecialist, avoiding the financial and time costs of unnecessary referrals and thus reduce the wait times for patients who do need subspecialty care visits.

Such efficiencies and cost savings are not only gained by the health care system, but also by patients and, in pediatrics in particular, the entire family. By one estimate illnesses for children in daycare can lead to 40% of parental missed workdays.[33] Services that can offer parents a means of obtaining medical care, without having to miss work, are thus a potentially huge benefit for families and society in terms of recovered workforce productivity. An urban pediatric telehealth program was shown to reduce the number of child absences caused by illness by more than 63%.[34] This telehealth program was well accepted by families, who most liked it for the convenience, time saved, and the ability to stay at work.[35] Such a program would thus allow parents to go to work, and reduce the burden on primary care clinics and EDs that are often used in these acute illnesses.

CHALLENGES TO THE ADOPTION OF TELEHEALTH

Despite the many potential benefits of telehealth within pediatrics, there are significant challenges that have hindered more widespread use. These include technological challenges, provider and patient concerns, financial barriers, credentialing barriers, and legal issues. These challenges are summarized in **Table 2**.

Technological Barriers

For telehealth to be practiced successfully, infrastructure must be in place at the consulting site and the sites requesting consultation. However, many communities do not have broadband connection of sufficient bandwidth to successfully conduct telehealth interactions.[20] This is particularly true in rural and underserved areas that are often most in need of telehealth to bridge critical gaps in access to specialty or critical care. In a pediatric cardiovascular home telehealth project, for example, researchers noted such variable access to quality landline and cell phones for data transmission that certain candidate subjects could not be enrolled because of lack

Table 2 Challenges to telehealth adoption	
Type of Challenge	**Specific Issues**
Technological barriers	• Lack of infrastructure, particularly in rural and underserved areas • Lack of high-quality systems to adequately convey imaging, like echocardiography and other radiologic testing
Provider concerns	• Lack of integration into current workflow, adding time to providers' already busy schedules • Resistance on the part of consulting providers "to step on the toes of others" • Resistance from community providers to being criticized or supervised • Discomfort with telehealth and associated technology because of lack of familiarity
Patient concerns	• Privacy concerns • Concerns about ability to properly use technology • Loss of face-to-face interactions with providers
Financial barriers	• Start-up and ongoing maintenance cost for technology, personnel, and training • Lack of clear and consistent reimbursement policies • Unclear return on investment • Misaligned incentives (ie, physicians would rather bring patients to their own institution, rather than spend extra time to keep a potential referral at a satellite site)
Credentialing and licensing barriers	• Many providers must get credentialed at all remote sites, which is a tremendous burden in terms of paperwork and time • State licensing requirements are highly variable and many states require providers to be licensed in any state in which they are providing telehealth consultation, not just their home state
Legal concerns	• Liability protections must be clear and protect providers at both sites

of stable telephone service.[36] Furthermore, for certain services to be useful, such as telehealth for radiology or echocardiography, the system quality must be high enough to ensure that images are able to be adequately interpreted by consulting specialists. Lack of access to high-quality equipment may make these services impossible to provide.

Provider Concerns

One of the biggest barriers to the use of telehealth has been resistance on the part of providers to embrace this technology in caring for patients. For many providers, telehealth is not easily integrated into routine workflow, adds extra time to their already busy schedules, and is perceived as often adding little benefit beyond a traditional telephone call.[37] From the community hospital physician perspective, many are distrustful of relying on consultants they do not know and do not want to feel supervised or criticized by having to reach out to others for help. Interestingly, consultant physicians in surveys have also expressed fears of being perceived as "stepping on toes" of community physicians.[38] In addition, when it comes to use of telehealth for sicker patients, many community providers believe it is safer to transfer those children to academic medical centers as quickly as possible and do not want to extend interactions with the hub sites or risk having a transfer denied.[37]

Lack of familiarity with telehealth and the equipment is another cause of physician resistance.[38] It is difficult to maintain provider competence with the equipment when volume is low. Fear of looking inept in front of physicians at other hospitals, and patients and families, makes providers who use the equipment infrequently even more hesitant to turn to telehealth.[37] Even among those providers who admit the overall benefit of using telehealth, many fail to see it as necessary or useful for their individual practice and therefore are slow to adopt it even in institutions promoting telehealth use.[38]

Patient Concerns

Compared with providers, patient and parent resistance to use of telehealth seems to be much less of a barrier. Nonetheless, there are important barriers for patients that need to be addressed. These include concerns about threats to privacy and security, concerns about the ability to use technology to appropriately communicate with providers, and loss of face-to-face interactions with physicians.[39] For providers using telehealth for home monitoring purposes, providers must ensure that patients and parents have access to necessary equipment, have the manual dexterity to adequately use that equipment, and have adequate health literacy and numeracy skills.[40]

Financial Barriers

There are several sources of financial barriers associated with telehealth. First, institutions or practices interested in engaging in telehealth must invest in the initial equipment costs to start a program. There are also continued costs of equipment maintenance, personnel training, and ongoing technical support. These costs may be particularly challenging for providers and hospitals in underserved and rural areas.[5]

Perhaps the largest financial barrier is the lack of clear and consistent reimbursement for telehealth and lack of return on investment. Currently, there is no universal reimbursement policy for telehealth encounters, and barriers exist for government and nongovernment insurers. As of 2007, a total of 35 states allowed for some reimbursement services, although not all states required reimbursement at the same rate as in-person encounters.[41] In 2010, the Center for Medicare and Medicaid Services established a consultation code for telehealth; however, its use is limited to hospitals outside of metropolitan areas.

Even when a payer may reimburse, some providers and programs fail to do so because of the time-consuming nature of the process.[37] Therefore, many telehealth programs rely on grant funding, which is typically time-limited and may not be sufficient for long-term sustainability. In addition, there is noticeable lack of evidence for return on investment. A recent systematic review found no evidence that telehealth interventions are cost effective compared with conventional health care.[42] However, methodologic issues may be hampering the ability to demonstrate cost savings in many studies.[20,42]

Misaligned incentives have also been reported as a barrier in studies of telehealth.[37] Although there may be benefits for the individual patient, such as getting to stay in a community hospital while avoiding transport to an academic medical center far from home, there may be no benefit, or in fact a disincentive, for the physicians involved. For example, a study of ED providers found that for hub hospitals, there is little incentive to help stabilize a patient in a community hospital. This results in extra work for the already busy provider being consulted and loss of a potential patient revenue for the hub hospital.[37]

Credentialing and Licensing Barriers

One of the biggest barriers reported in the literature to telehealth is the credentialing process for providers.[20,37,38,41] The credentialing process for an individual hospital often involves tremendous amounts of paperwork and can take months to go through. For a provider at a hub hospital, completing paperwork for each potential spoke hospital at which he or she will provide telehealth consultation can therefore involve a huge amount of redundant, time-consuming work. In 2011, Center for Medicare and Medicaid Services and The Joint Commission allowed for "credentialing by proxy" to allow spoke hospitals to rely on the credentialing decisions of the hub hospital. However, many community hospitals refuse to do so out of fear of liability concerns, and certain states have opted not to allow credentialing by proxy.[43]

There is also significant variation with regard to licensure requirements for physicians practicing telehealth. Licensure is performed at a state level, and generally the place of service is the location in which a patient has a face-to-face encounter with a clinical provider. Whether a provider requires full licensure in all states in which they serve as a consultant, licensing only from their home state, or a special telehealth license is highly variable. Currently, only 33 states have specifically addressed telehealth practice across state lines, eight authorizing a "special purpose" license for cross-state telehealth practice. Twenty-one states require full licensure for out-of-state physicians providing telehealth consultation services.[44]

Legal Concerns

There are several legal issues raised by telehealth, which are of significant concern to many providers and organizations. One issue is with regard to medicolegal liability. For example, clear liability protections must be in place at both sites to protect providers consulting on patients remotely, and to protect those providers following the remote consultants' advice. Telehealth is a middle ground between face-to-face encounters and telephone encounters, and in theory care should be improved over telephone encounters because of the improved ability of the consulting physician to visualize the patient. However, research on telephone malpractice cases has found them to be extremely costly with regard to settlements, and result in significant morbidity and even mortality—indeed, death was the most common injury, occurring in 44% of claims reviewed.[45] Understandably, providers and organizations may be wary of the medicolegal liability dangers, particularly if there is concern about the return on investment. It is also unclear what might happen in the case of technology failure.

SUMMARY

The role of telehealth technology in the delivery of pediatric health care is only expected to increase in the coming years. Although there are currently major regulatory barriers that still need to be overcome, the support for telehealth in legislation, such as the ACA, suggests that the government sees this as part of the future of medicine. To continue to advance telehealth, patients and providers must argue for certain policies and reforms to address the barriers discussed in this article. This has been underscored in the recent AAP policy statement on use of telehealth.[5] Specific recommendations include the following:

- Efforts to continue to grow and expand telehealth services should be supported with the goal of maintaining care, whenever possible, within the context of the PCMH
- More robust funding mechanisms supporting telehealth services must be developed, including state and federal funding, private investment, and grant opportunities

- Training in telehealth should be formalized into medical school and graduate medical education programs
- Adequate payment mechanisms that support the time and effort of referring and participating facilities must be established
- Policies regulating licensure and credentialing must be developed that reduce the burden on individual providers and organizations attempting to engage in telehealth services
- Rigorous research should be conducted on the use of telehealth services to understand its most effective uses, including the potential for increasing cost-effective care

By developing health policy in this arena, the potential of telehealth technology can be better fulfilled. Use of telehealth services can help transform health care delivery within pediatrics, importantly addressing critical gaps in access for rural and underserved populations, and those with more complex health needs. The growth of patient interest in telehealth, along with improving access to the Internet in homes and via mobile devices, make the time perfect for using innovations and advances to help providers engage with their patients and other providers in new ways to deliver medical care outside the office.

REFERENCES

1. Public law 111-148. The patient protection and affordable care act. 2010. Available at: http://www.gpo.gov/fdsys/pkg/PLAW-111publ148/pdf/PLAW-111publ148.pdf. Accessed August 8, 2015.
2. Institute of Medicine. The role of telehealth in an evolving health care environment: workshop summary. Washington, DC: National Academies Press (US); 2012.
3. Modahl M. Telehealth index: 2015 consumer survey. 2015. Available at: http://info.americanwell.com/telehealth-index-2015-consumer-survey. Accessed August 10, 2015.
4. Emerman E. Health care benefits cost increases to hold steady in 2016, national business group on health survey finds. National Business Group on Health; 2015. Available at: http://www.businessgrouphealth.org/pressroom/pressRelease.cfm?ID=263. Accessed August 13, 2015.
5. Committee on Pediatric Workforce. The use of telemedicine to address access and physician workforce shortages. Pediatrics 2015;136(1):202–9.
6. Zundel KM. Telemedicine: history, applications, and impact on librarianship. Bull Med Libr Assoc 1996;84(1):71–9.
7. Institute of Medicine (US), Field MJ. Telemedicine: a guide to assessing telecommunications in health care. Washington, DC: National Academies Press; 1996.
8. What is telehealth? How is telehealth different from telemedicine? HealthITgov. Available at: http://www.healthit.gov/providers-professionals/faqs/what-telehealth-how-telehealth-different-telemedicine. Accessed July 10, 2015.
9. What is Telemedicine? Available at: http://www.americantelemed.org/about-telemedicine/what-is-telemedicine. Accessed August 14, 2015.
10. Allely EB. Synchronous and asynchronous telemedicine. J Med Syst 1995;19(3):207–12.
11. Hersh WR, Hickam DH, Severance SM, et al. Diagnosis, access and outcomes: update of a systematic review of telemedicine services. J Telemed Telecare 2006;12(Suppl 2):S3–31.

12. Vital Wave Consulting. mHealth for development: the opportunity of mobile technology for healthcare in the developing world. Washington, DC; Berkshire (United Kingdom): UN Foundation-Vodafone Foundation Partnership; 2009.

13. McConnochie KM, Conners GP, Brayer AF, et al. Effectiveness of telemedicine in replacing in-person evaluation for acute childhood illness in office settings. Telemed J E Health 2006;12(3):308–16.

14. Sable CA, Cummings SD, Pearson GD, et al. Impact of telemedicine on the practice of pediatric cardiology in community hospitals. Pediatrics 2002;109(1):E3.

15. Marcin JP, Ellis J, Mawis R, et al. Using telemedicine to provide pediatric subspecialty care to children with special health care needs in an underserved rural community. Pediatrics 2004;113(1 Pt 1):1–6.

16. Richter GM, Sun G, Lee TC, et al. Speed of telemedicine vs ophthalmoscopy for retinopathy of prematurity diagnosis. Am J Ophthalmol 2009;148(1): 136–42.e2.

17. Reese RM, Jamison R, Wendland M, et al. Evaluating interactive videoconferencing for assessing symptoms of autism. Telemed J E Health 2013;19(9):671–7.

18. Fogel AL, Teng JMC. Pediatric teledermatology: a survey of usage, perspectives, and practice. Pediatr Dermatol 2015;32(3):363–8.

19. Mair F, Whitten P. Systematic review of studies of patient satisfaction with telemedicine. BMJ 2000;320(7248):1517–20.

20. Burke BL, Hall RW, Section on Telehealth Care. Telemedicine: pediatric applications. Pediatrics 2015;136(1):e293–308.

21. Children's Hospital Association. Childrenshospitals.org; 2014. Available at: https://www.childrenshospitals.org/About-Us/About-Childrens-Hospitals. Accessed August 12, 2015.

22. Ray KN, Demirci JR, Bogen DL, et al. Optimizing telehealth strategies for subspecialty care: recommendations from rural pediatricians. Telemed J E Health 2015; 21(8):622–9.

23. Garingo A, Friedlich P, Chavez T, et al. "Tele-rounding" with a remotely controlled mobile robot in the neonatal intensive care unit. J Telemed Telecare 2015;1–7. http://dx.doi.org/10.1177/1357633X15589478.

24. Marcin JP, Nesbitt TS, Kallas HJ, et al. Use of telemedicine to provide pediatric critical care inpatient consultations to underserved rural Northern California. J Pediatr 2004;144(3):375–80.

25. Ellenby MS, Marcin JP. The role of telemedicine in pediatric critical care. Crit Care Clin 2015;31(2):275–90.

26. Dharmar M, Kuppermann N, Romano PS, et al. Telemedicine consultations and medication errors in rural emergency departments. Pediatrics 2013;132(6): 1090–7.

27. Hernandez M, Hojman N, Sadorra C, et al. Pediatric critical care telemedicine program: a single institution review. Telemed J E Health 2015. http://dx.doi.org/10.1089/tmj.2015.0043.

28. Ekeland AG, Bowes A, Flottorp S. Effectiveness of telemedicine: a systematic review of reviews. Int J Med Inform 2010;79(11):736–71.

29. Gonzalez-Espada WJ, Hall-Barrow J, Hall RW, et al. Achieving success connecting academic and practicing clinicians through telemedicine. Pediatrics 2009; 123(3):e476–83.

30. Marcin JP, Nesbitt TS, Struve S, et al. Financial benefits of a pediatric intensive care unit-based telemedicine program to a rural adult intensive care unit: impact of keeping acutely ill and injured children in their local community. Telemed J E Health 2004;10(Suppl 2):S-1–5.

31. Mahnke CB, Jordan CP, Bergvall E, et al. The Pacific Asynchronous TeleHealth (PATH) system: review of 1,000 pediatric teleconsultations. Telemed J E Health 2011;17(1):35–9.
32. Smith AK, White DB, Arnold RM. Uncertainty — the other side of prognosis. N Engl J Med 2013;368(26):2448–50.
33. Bell DM, Gleiber DW, Mercer AA, et al. Illness associated with child day care: a study of incidence and cost. Am J Public Health 1989;79(4):479–84.
34. McConnochie KM. Telemedicine reduces absence resulting from illness in urban child care: evaluation of an innovation. Pediatrics 2005;115(5):1273–82.
35. McConnochie KM, Wood NE, Herendeen NE, et al. Telemedicine in urban and suburban childcare and elementary schools lightens family burdens. Telemed J E Health 2010;16(5):533–42.
36. Black AK, Sadanala UK, Mascio CE, et al. Challenges in implementing a pediatric cardiovascular home telehealth project. Telemed J E Health 2014;20(9):858–67.
37. Uscher-Pines L, Kahn JM. Barriers and facilitators to pediatric emergency telemedicine in the United States. Telemed J E Health 2014;20(11):990–6.
38. Rogove HJ, McArthur D, Demaerschalk BM, et al. Barriers to telemedicine: survey of current users in acute care units. Telemed J E Health 2012;18(1):48–53.
39. Sanders C, Rogers A, Bowen R, et al. Exploring barriers to participation and adoption of telehealth and telecare within the whole system demonstrator trial: a qualitative study. BMC Health Serv Res 2012;12(1):220.
40. Kaufman DR, Starren J, Patel VL, et al. A cognitive framework for understanding barriers to the productive use of a diabetes home telemedicine system. AMIA Annu Symp Proc 2003;356–60.
41. Soares NS, Langkamp DL. Telehealth in developmental-behavioral pediatrics. J Dev Behav Pediatr 2012;33(8):656–65.
42. Mistry H. Systematic review of studies of the cost-effectiveness of telemedicine and telecare. Changes in the economic evidence over twenty years. J Telemed Telecare 2012;18(1):1–6.
43. Reimbursement. The Robert J. Waters center for telehealth and e-health law. Available at: http://ctel.org/expertise/reimbursement. Accessed July 17, 2015.
44. Center for telehealth and e-health law. The Robert J. Waters Center for telehealth and e-health law. Available at: http://ctel.org. Accessed July 16, 2015.
45. Katz HP, Kaltsounis D, Halloran L, et al. Patient safety and telephone medicine. J Gen Intern Med 2008;23(5):517–22.

Index

Note: Page numbers of article titles are in **boldface** type.

A

Access to care, telehealth for, 370
Accreditation Council for Graduate Medical Education, 304, 306–307
Acute Care Model, 270–271
Adult health outcomes, pediatric care impact on, 224
Adverse outcomes, prediction of, 260–261
Advocacy, importance of, 224
Affordable Care Act
    costs and, 330, 332
    telehealth and, 368
Agency for Health Care Research and Quality, **239–249**, 284
American Board of Pediatrics, quality improvement training and, 270
American College of Graduate Medical Education, quality improvement courses of, 270
American Medical Informatics Association, 365
American Nurses Association, 336
Analytics, **357–366**
    advanced, 360–361
    architectural framework in, 359
    challenges in, 364
    data scientists role in, 360
    decision support and, 358–359
    definition of, 358
    in clinical decision support, 360–361
    in hospital operation, 360
Architectural framework, in analytics, 359
Asthma, inpatient care for, 288
Asynchronous telehealth, 368–369

B

Before-after technology interventions, research based on, 254
Bell-shaped curves, 350–352
Benchmarking, for safety and quality improvement, **239–249**
Best Evidence Medical Education review, 307–308
Best practice alerts, for emergency care, 275
Big data
    for predictive analytics, **357–366**
    genomics and, 361–363
    in intensive care unit, 296–297
Biostatistics, 350–352
Board certification, 364–365
Boston Children's Hospital, 310

Pediatr Clin N Am 63 (2016) 379–387
http://dx.doi.org/10.1016/S0031-3955(16)00023-7
0031-3955/16/$ – see front matter © 2016 Elsevier Inc. All rights reserved.
pediatric.theclinics.com

Moving?

Make sure your subscription moves with you!

To notify us of your new address, find your **Clinics Account Number** (located on your mailing label above your name), and contact customer service at:

Email: journalscustomerservice-usa@elsevier.com

800-654-2452 (subscribers in the U.S. & Canada)
314-447-8871 (subscribers outside of the U.S. & Canada)

Fax number: 314-447-8029

Elsevier Health Sciences Division
Subscription Customer Service
3251 Riverport Lane
Maryland Heights, MO 63043

*To ensure uninterrupted delivery of your subscription, please notify us at least 4 weeks in advance of move.